LOVE YOUR SKIN

YOUR

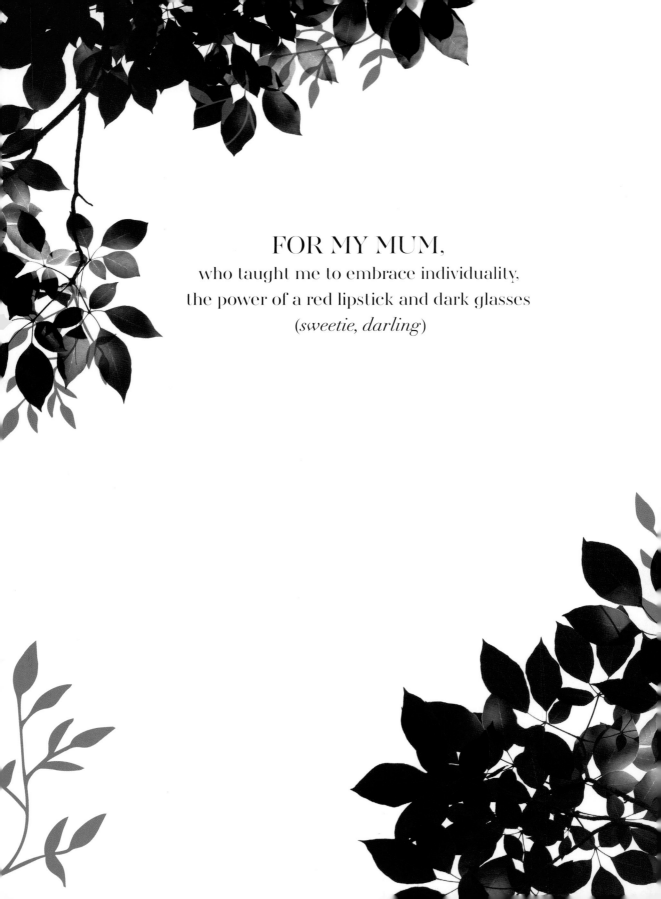

FOR MY MUM,
who taught me to embrace individuality,
the power of a red lipstick and dark glasses
(*sweetie, darling*)

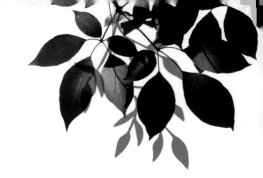

the
ULTIMATE
guide to
a glowing
complexion

LOVE
YOUR
SKIN

Abigail James

Photography by Jenni Hare

Kyle Books

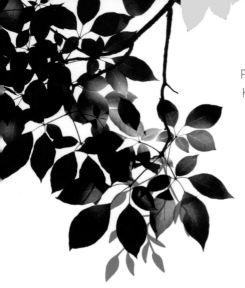

First published in Great Britain in 2017 by
Kyle Books, an imprint of Kyle Cathie Ltd
192–198 Vauxhall Bridge Road
London SW1V 1DX
general.enquiries@kylebooks.com
www.kylebooks.co.uk

10 9 8 7 6 5 4 3 2 1

ISBN 978 0 85783 414 0

Editor: Judith Hannam
Editorial Assisant: Hannah Coughlin
Copy Editor: Liz Murray
Art direction & design: Nikki Dupin
Photographer: Jenni Hare
Hair and makeup: Lica Fensome (and Nigel Barnes page 81)
Stylist: Andie Redman
Production: Lisa Pinnell
Models: Adena Wallingford, Bruna Vehlho, Emma Barley,
Grace Cotton, Mariia Babikova, Sylvia Flote, Gabriella Riggon-Allen

A Cataloguing in Publication record for this title is available
from the British Library.

Colour reproduction by ALTA London
Printed and bound in China by 1010 International Printing Ltd.

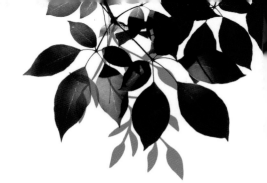

contents

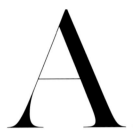A career in the health and beauty industry wasn't my first choice. I wanted to be a jewellery designer, though I began my working life alongside my father in the family food company. It wasn't until I had my first child at the age of 23 and found myself suffering from post-natal depression that I decided to take stock and retrain as a beauty therapist. Juggling motherhood and education was never going to be easy, but learning about the intricacies of the face, the body, about skincare ingredients, ancient therapies and futuristic science made the hard work worthwhile and I knew I had found my true calling.

Newly qualified, I began building up my own client base in the spas, salons and private homes of the Cotswolds. Since then, my passion for helping people achieve their best skin and health whatever their age has never left me. Nor has my thirst for learning. I've spent the past decade expanding my knowledge with continued study of a wide variety of methods for the face and body. I've worked with some of the most respected skin and spa brands designing treatments and also mentored therapists for some of the world's most beautiful hotels and retreats, dipping into nutrition, massage, yoga, Ayurveda and acupressure.

This journey has really formed my philosophy about looking good and feeling vibrant – that healthy, glowing skin isn't achieved by the latest 'miracle' cream or 'super' ingredient, but by a balance of well-chosen products and treatments, exercise, stress management techniques, an awareness of our hormonal cycle and, of course, food. So all that time spent working with my father wasn't wasted!

Whatever your budget, lifestyle, age, ethnicity or skin type you can achieve a complexion you can be proud of, so long as you learn to understand and respond to your skin as it changes throughout life. This is why I've included chapters on all of the above topics, sharing my years of experience and insider tips to help you discover how to get the best from your skin. I want to encourage you to throw away the notion that looking after your skin and face is a luxury or a treat. Giving attention to something we look at daily and engage with others by isn't vanity, but an essential confidence boost, plus it makes us happy.

I hope you'll enjoy practising the techniques displayed and learning more about what might work for you and your skin, whipping up your own kitchen cupboard beauty remedies in the process. After many years of seeing clients, I know that the link between our skin, our identity and our sense of self-worth is inextricable. Which is why I hope you'll grow to trust this book, just as you would a great friend.

Wishing you the very best of luck in discovering your most vibrant, confident beautiful self.

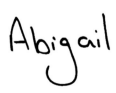

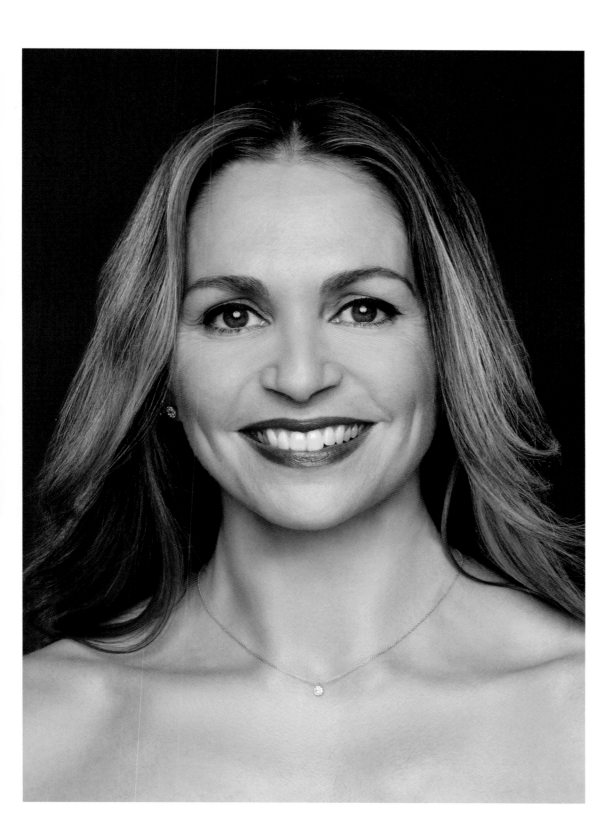

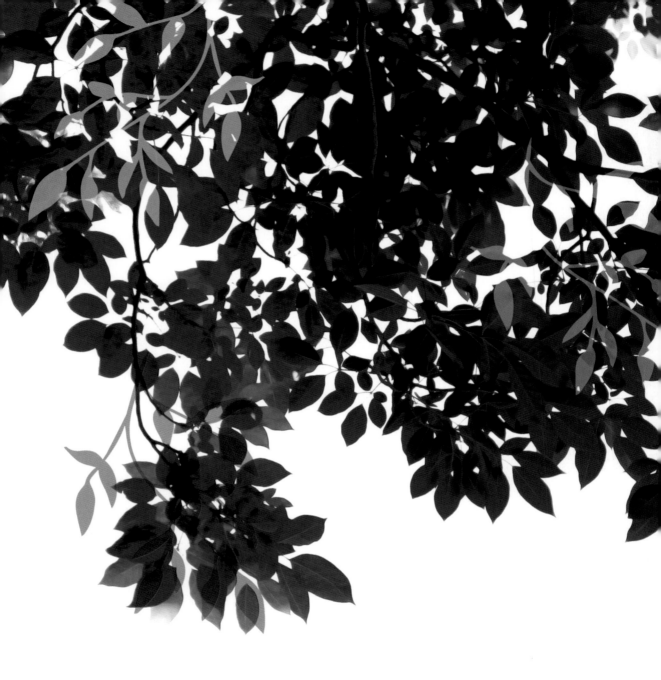

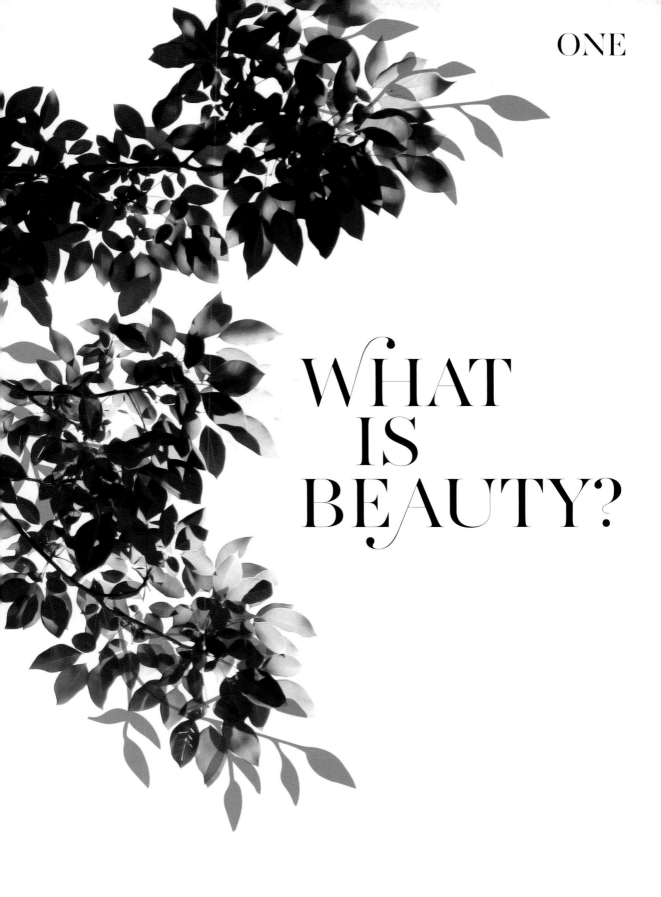

ONE

WHAT IS BEAUTY?

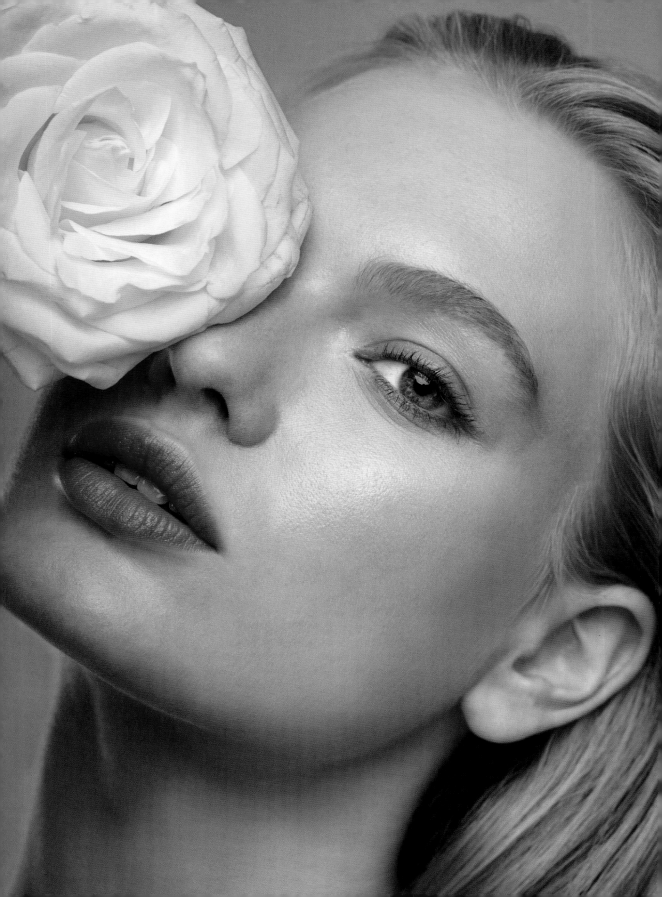

"*Beauty* is not about a face full of make-up, beauty is an *attitude*"

THE BEAUTY *of* CONFIDENCE

> The true beauty in a woman is reflected in her soul. It is the caring that she lovingly gives, the passion that she shows. The beauty of a woman grows with the passing years.
>
> AUDREY HEPBURN

Beauty counters can be alluring yet daunting places. Like moths to a flame, we're drawn in by the beautiful packaging, the latest 'miracle' product, the perfect red lipstick. My introduction to them came in my early teens. I felt so grown up. The bottle was pink, the cream inside smelt sweet and floral – and it gave me a severe rash for days! Despite this, I've since enjoyed a lasting love affair with the skincare industry.

The desire to feel attractive is hardwired into us all. It's a force of nature – and it's what drives humans to reproduce. We want to look forever young and beautiful, yet in the words of one of my own all-time favourite beauty icons, Audrey Hepburn: The true beauty in a woman is reflected in her soul. It is the caring that she lovingly gives, the passion that she shows. The beauty of a woman grows with the passing years.

With the right products, treatments and health we can all have great skin. The problem is that in an era driven by social media, 'selfies' and airbrushing, our expectations have lost touch with reality. We want to look eternally youthful, to turn back time and shun age – as if it's something of which to be ashamed.

There's something undeniably beautiful about a truly confident person. Even if they don't have an archetypal symmetry, they radiate something powerfully magnetic. An international study of 8,000 women across 16 countries revealed that women's desire to boost their self-confidence now equals their wish to change their outer appearance. For many of us, though, achieving inner confidence is difficult. We are bombarded by professional and personal demands, all day, every day. In the background to all this noise is our own inner voice, which is often our harshest critic. It whispers cruel, negative judgements about our appearance so frequently that we start to believe them.

By turning this habit on its head and making these thoughts positive, we can start to think more appreciatively of ourselves. Our inner voice talks to us more than anybody else, so make sure that what you say to yourself is kind.

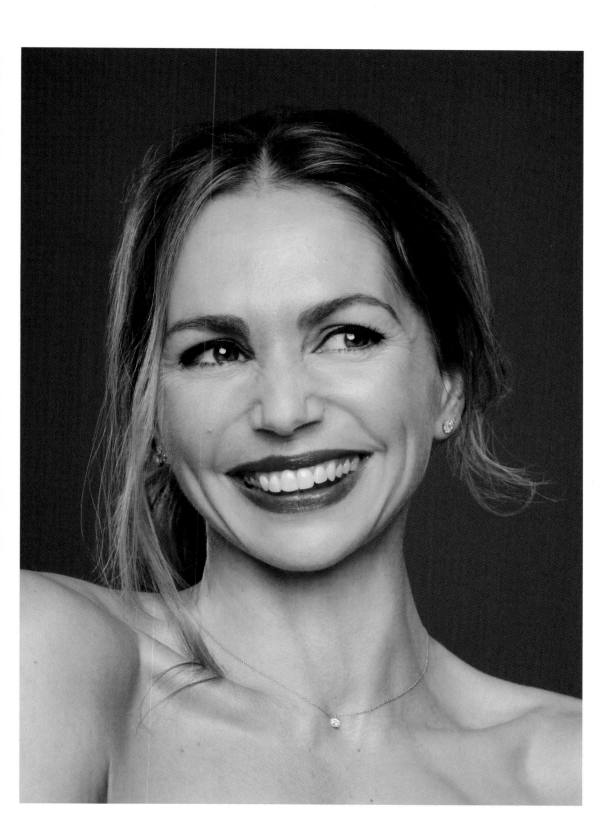

How *the* skin works . . .

The skin is our largest organ and many of us take it for granted. Knowing how it works will help you better understand it and to make better product and lifestyle choices. Most importantly, skin makes us look the way we do. It tells the story of our lives, reveals our joy and our pain. But beyond aesthetics, skin also has several vital functions to fulfil, including:

1. PROTECTION:
it acts as a barrier against external environmental damage.

2. SENSATION:
it contains a variety of nerve endings that react to heat, cold, touch, pressure, vibration and tissue injury.

3. HEAT REGULATION:
it contains blood vessels, which allow precise control of energy and heat loss through dilation and constriction.

4. CONTROL OF EVAPORATION:
it provides an almost dry and impermeable barrier to fluid loss.

5. STORAGE AND SYNTHESIS:
it acts as a storage centre for lipids and water, as well as a means of synthesising vitamin D.

6. EXCRETION:
the production of sweat cools the skin through evaporation. Sweat also contains urea, so acts as a means of removing waste substances from the body.

7. ABSORPTION:
oxygen, nitrogen and carbon dioxide can diffuse into the skin in small amounts. In addition, medicine can be administered through the skin by ointments or by means of an adhesive patch, such as a nicotine patch.

8. WATER RESISTANCE:
the skin acts as a water-resistant barrier so essential nutrients aren't washed out of the body.

9. AESTHETICS AND COMMUNICATION:
others see our skin and can assess our mood, health and attractiveness.

10. SKIN IS ALSO CONNECTED TO OUR EMOTIONS:
when we love how our skin looks, we feel confident and happy.

Did *you* know . . .

- The skin makes up approximately 12–15 percent of our total body weight.

- The average person has 20,000sq cm of skin and 300 million skin cells.

- Humans shed about 600,000 particles of skin every hour – about 700g a year.

- By 70 years of age, the average person will have lost 48kg of skin.

- Each 3sq cm of skin has approximately ten hairs, 15 sebaceous glands, 100 sweat glands and 100cm of tiny blood vessels.

- There are 72km of nerves in the skin of a human being.

- It is about 1mm in thickness over most of the body but in areas where it's at its thinnest such as the eyelids, it's only about 0.5mm. Skin is thickest on the soles of the feet and palms of our hands. In these places, it can be up to 1.5mm thick.

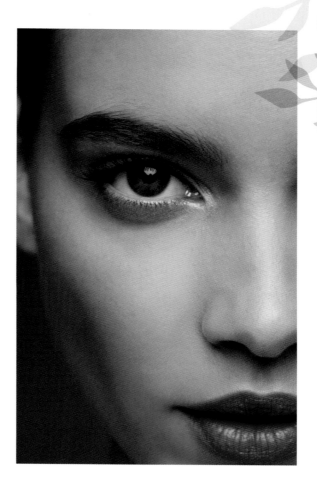

The skin cycle

As we get older, the rate at which our skin cells renew is greatly reduced, causing dullness, dryness and the visible signs of age. Put simply, when we age, our skin cells aren't as energetic as they once were! For this reason, it's best to give a product at least a month to work and deliver results. Using exfoliants, peels and ingredients that boost your skin cell turnover will allow newer, fresher skin to be visible on the surface.

the ANATOMY *of* SKIN

Skin is made up of three main layers:
the *epidermis*, the *dermis* and the *subcutaneous* layer

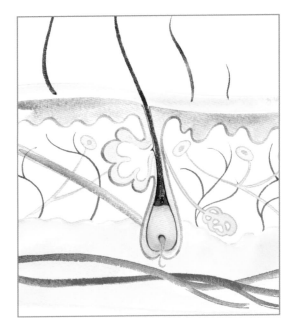

"

Beauty is so much more than skin deep. Our skin reflects our inner health and happiness.

- **THE EPIDERMIS** – the barrier layer
At approximately 0.1mm thick, this outermost layer forms a protective, waterproof barrier over the whole body. It contains no blood vessels but is home to pigment and proteins. Skin cells move up to this layer from beneath and are shed on a daily basis. This exfoliation process takes around 28 days in young, healthy skin but slows with age and is also affected by diet, hormones, sun exposure, smoking and physical exercise.

- **THE DERMIS** – the strength layer
This middle layer contains blood vessels, nerves, hair follicles and oil glands, as well as a tough supportive mass of connective tissues called collagen and elastin. These two types of protein give skin its strength and youthful elasticity.

- **THE SUBCUTANEOUS LAYER**
– the cushioning layer
This contains sweat glands, some hair follicles, blood vessels and fat, and gives the skin its natural plumpness. It's made up of loose connective tissue and fat cells that insulate and protect your internal organs. Connective tissue has collagen fibres to give support and elastin fibres to provide flexibility and strength. Collagen is a protein that makes up 70 per cent of the building blocks within our skin. The body is constantly renewing its collagen, yet the cells that produce collagen fibres (known as fibroblasts) become less active with age. Over time, collagen fibres get thicker and easier to break. After the age of twenty-five, the amount produced reduces by about 1 per cent a year.

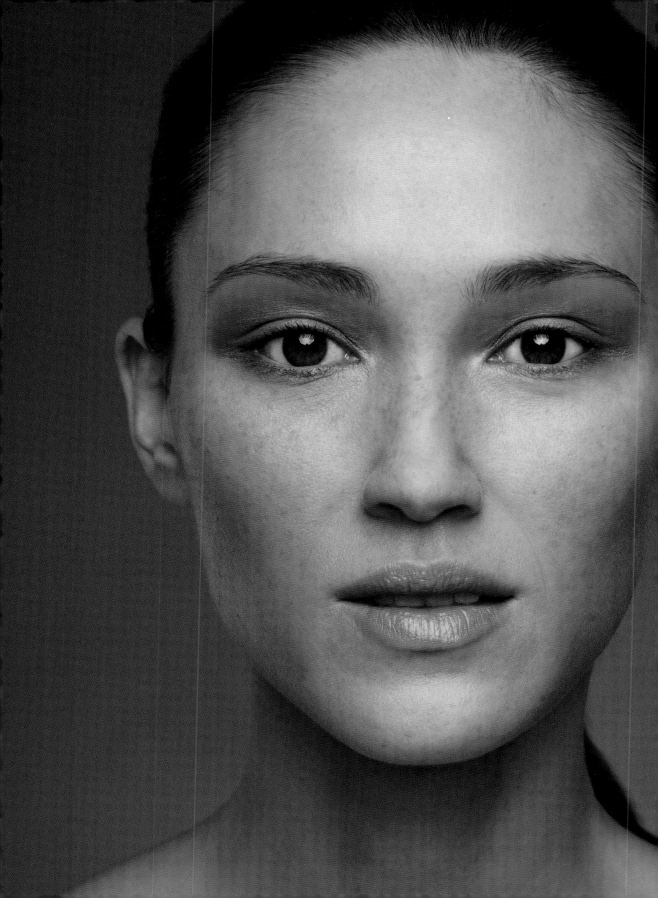

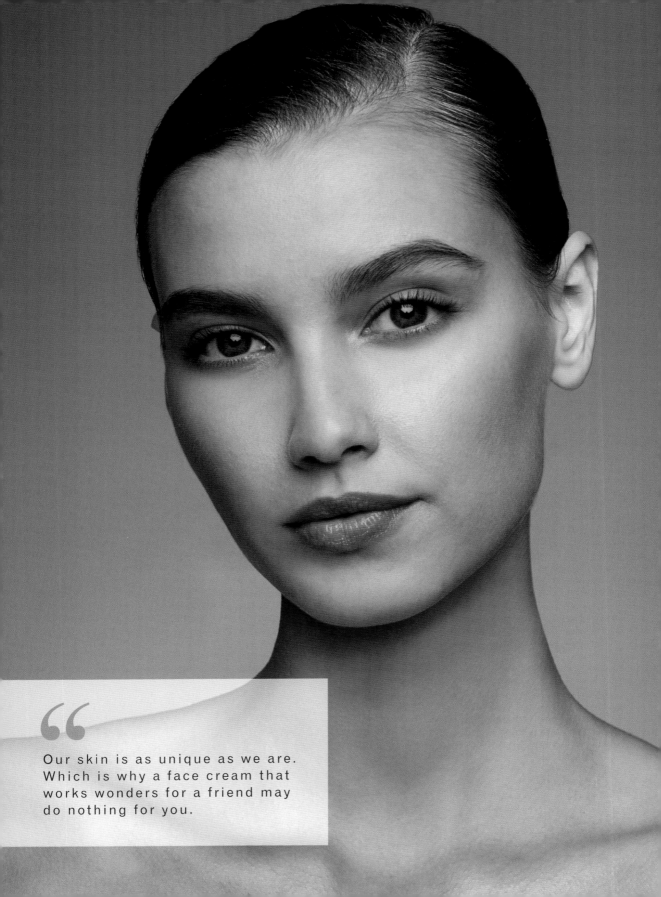

“

Our skin is as unique as we are.
Which is why a face cream that
works wonders for a friend may
do nothing for you.

Your SKIN'S FAMILY TREE

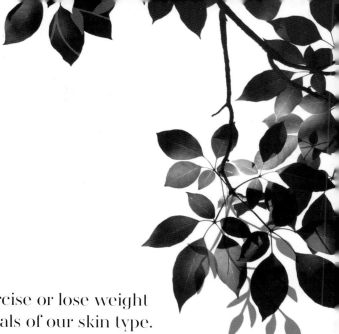

We *can* change our body shape – exercise or lose weight – but we *can't* change the fundamentals of our skin type.

Our skin is as unique as we are. Which is why a face cream that works wonders for a friend may do nothing for you. Or why the slightest bit of stress causes your skin to break out but your friend, who is a bigger stress bunny, has flawless skin. Genetics, ethnicity, diet and where you live all play a role, and can be divided into two basic factors: intrinsic ageing and extrinsic ageing.

INTRINSIC AGEING is what we're born with. To some extent, we are pre-wired to age at a certain rate throughout our lifetime. The pace at which our production of collagen and elastin declines and at which we develop lines, wrinkles, hooded eyelids and sunken cheeks is inherited from our parents and the generations of family members before them.

EXTRINSIC AGEING is affected by external lifestyle factors – the climate we live in, our sun exposure, stress levels, diet and consumption of alcohol and sugar, and whether we smoke or take the contraceptive pill.

EXTRINSIC FACTORS

- **location**

I'm a country girl born and bred. I started as a skin therapist in the Cotswolds, then later began seeing clients in London. I was able to see how location affects the skin. In the countryside, I'd see broken capillaries, sensitivity, rosacea and skin weathered by a life spent outdoors. In London, my clients' skin was more congested and adult acne was a concern for many women. Pollution, stress, fast food eaten on the go and late nights all take a toll.

- **climate**

A dry climate results in the skin becoming drier and prone to sensitivity, and fine lines will develop earlier. In colder climates, skin can become chapped. In humid conditions, skin retains more moisture, but this can exacerbate problems with oily skin as you sweat more, and pores become blocked so breakouts occur.

HORMONES

Hormones are intrinsic factors, but they are hugely affected by extrinsic considerations. Part of the endocrine system, they play a vital role in the way our skin looks and feels. When our hormones are balanced we feel happy and healthy. Physically, we have vibrant skin, a good sex drive, regular monthly cycles, shiny hair and a steady body weight.

Most of us think of the male and female hormones – testosterone, oestrogen and progesterone – when we hear the word 'hormones', but we have many others. I like to imagine that they're all lined up in test tubes, each filled with the precise amount of hormone needed to maintain balance within the body. If one gets spilled, or another gets topped up, all of the others have to fight to retain overall balance. This internal struggle is what dictates the condition of our skin. Each of these hormones has a different impact upon the skin:

- **OESTROGEN:** the female hormone, which makes women's skin dewy, hydrated, plump and youthful. The skin ages as oestrogen levels drop.

- **TESTOSTERONE:** the male hormone that results in oilier, thicker skin and stimulates collagen production.

- **ANDROGENS:** are made of many male hormones but women have them too. They stimulate collagen production and make the skin stronger and oilier. These play a role in acne breakouts.

An important gland that affects the skin is the thyroid. This makes two hormones that affect brain development, breathing, bone health, body temperature, weight gain or loss, muscle strength and metabolism. If your thyroid is overactive, you can become warm, sweaty and flushed. If it's underactive, your skin may become dry.

If you have an underlying hormone imbalance, there may not be a magic cream or potion that will fix your skin; however, there will be some lifestyles, treatments and products that will help you support your skin to keep it on track. Common symptoms that indicate that your hormones might be out of whack include:

- Feeling lethargic
- Thinning hair
- Loss of sex drive
- Skin breakouts
- Weight gain
- Mood swings
- Mental fogginess
- Sleeplessness
- Anxiety and feeling low
- Hot flushes and night sweats

12 ways to rebalance *your* hormones

1. Reduce toxins in the form of pesticides and certain plastics and household chemicals. Bisphenol is a chemical commonly used in water bottles and food packaging. Phthalates and PVC are found in some cosmetics and hair products.

2. Eat organic where possible. I realise that it costs more, but if your body is showing signs of toxic overload it might be an investment worth trying.

3. Cook food at home rather than grabbing pre-packed foods on the go.

4. Increase your intake of magnesium. The best way to get magnesium is topically, so try an oil or a spray.

5. Use a water filter.

6. Support your liver. As a key elimination organ responsible for metabolising hormones, it's crucial that you keep it healthy. Do this by eating foods such as broccoli, kale, cabbage, brussels sprouts, turnips and leafy greens.

7. Cut down on coffee. It tends to send hormones haywire, so switch to herbal teas. If you still crave the taste of coffee, try decaffeinated or roasted dandelion tea. And if you must have a coffee, drink it before 3pm as it will reduce its the impact. Always follow it with a large glass of water to help flush it through your body.

8. Consider cutting out alcohol. It puts extra stress on your liver and imbalances blood-sugar levels. Try not to drink on an empty stomach and match each glass of wine with one of water. Taking a vitamin B supplement the morning after will help your liver's detoxification process. Chlorella is also a fantastic supplement to counterbalance the harmful effects of alcohol.

9. Avoid bad fats. Sunflower, corn and peanut oils are often included within processed foods. These are what I call 'bad fats'. Foods high in omega-3 fats are 'good fats' that fight inflammation. These can be found in flax and chia seeds, cod liver oil and sea buckthorn.

10. Be wary of phytoestrogens. These are naturally occurring substances in plants that have hormone-like activity, found in foods such as soy. While some soy is good for us, too much can prevent the body from processing iodine, which is stored in the thyroid gland, breasts and ovaries and responsible for cell metabolism and supporting hormone balance.

11. Don't exercise to excess. I'm not suggesting that you give up your gym membership and your fitness routine. Yet very strenuous cardio, repeated day in day out, can unbalance your hormones and affect your menstrual cycle. So everything in balance! Mix it up with some lighter swimming, walking, Pilates or yoga.

12. Take supplements of iodine, a trace mineral most of us are deficient in, found in seafood and seaweed; vitamin D3, found in cod liver oil; magnesium, which supports hundreds of processes in the body and often contributes to better sleep, and milk thistle, good for supporting the liver.

Healthy hormone shopping list

- ✓ Chia seeds
- ✓ Flaxseed
- ✓ Sunflower seeds
- ✓ Sesame seeds
- ✓ Pine nuts
- ✓ Pistachios
- ✓ Eggs – including the yolks
- ✓ Oily fish
- ✓ Almonds

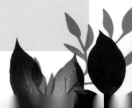

HAVING *the* RIGHT BALANCE *of* ANTIOXIDANTS & FREE RADICALS

Free radicals are unstable molecules found everywhere – in the air, in our bodies and in the materials around us.

Pollution, sunlight and smoking trigger the production of more free radicals. They attach themselves to healthy cells in an attempt to make themselves more stable. As a result, the healthy cells become free radicals too. Our bodies need some free radicals as they play a vital part in fighting bacteria, but when we have more free radicals than antioxidants, we suffer oxidative stress, which causes cells to become damaged. To counteract oxidative stress, our body produces an army of antioxidants. I like to imagine these as calm, mediator cells. They bring free radicals back into balance, without being compromised themselves. For optimum health – and beautiful skin – it's essential to have a diet high in antioxidants.

GETTING ENOUGH ANTIOXIDANTS

Vitamins A, C, E, folic acid, beta-carotene and phytochemicals such as carotenoids, flavanoids, allyl sulfides and polyphenols are all antioxidants that benefit the skin. Most natural whole foods, such as whole grains, fruits and vegetables, contain phytochemicals, whereas processed or refined foods contain little to none. Modern-day farming methods mean that the plants we consume aren't as packed with antioxidants as they were just a few decades ago, so you may need to gain extra nutrients and support from supplements. Antioxidants are widely used within skincare and each one has a different benefit. All plants have some antioxidant content, so it's about utilising those with the highest amounts and also how the cream or serum is formulated to deliver them into the skin. Some of my favourite topical antioxidants are vitamin C, vitamin E, resveratrol, retinol and green tea.

The 70–30 rule

If for 70 per cent of the time you nurture your skin and body with healthy food, moderate exercise and good skincare, the remaining 30 per cent you can let your hair down. Have that glass of wine, enjoy chocolate – your skin won't fall off if you leave your make-up on for one night. Striving for unattainable perfection merely perpetuates the cycle of negativity.

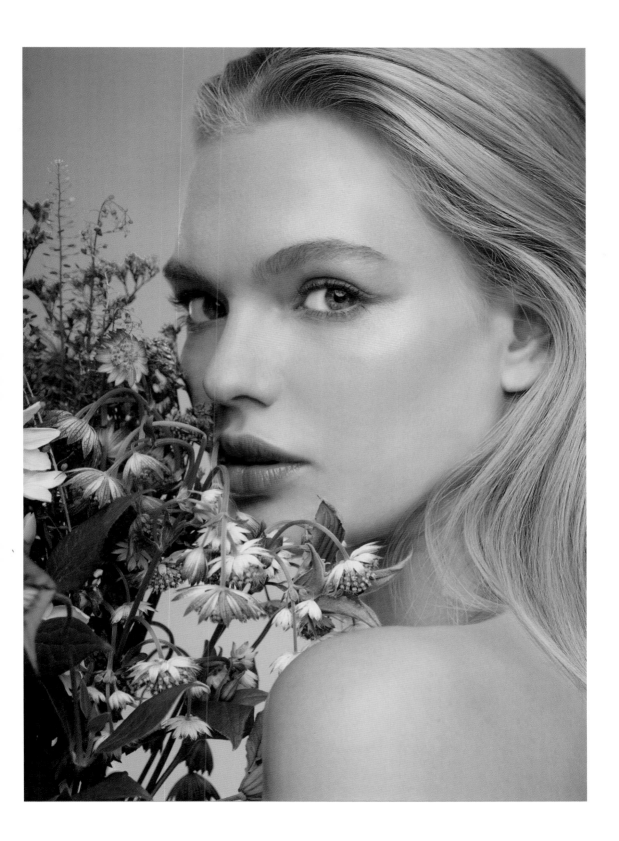

WATER, WATER, EVERYWHERE

We're all aware that drinking more water will benefit our skin, but *why?*

Did *you* know . . .

- Cells are 70 per cent water so need it to function properly. Healthy cells result in a more rapid renewal rate and a more glowing complexion.

- A well-hydrated cell is plump and softens the appearance of fine lines.

- Drinking water helps flush out toxins and keep the skin looking fresh. Try starting each day with a 2-litre bottle and ensure you drink half before lunch and the other half through the afternoon.

- If you drink your daily quota in one go, your body will simply wee the excess out rather than use it. If, however, you stagger your intake, your body will absorb and use it. The body will naturally hydrate the vital internal organs first, as it's how the body survives. The skin is the last organ to become hydrated.

- Drinking eight glasses a day should be a minimum. How many you need each day may vary. Have you had five coffees? Did you do a sweaty commute? A gym class? Are you taking medication? Going through the menopause? Have you had sex? All these things will impact on how much extra hydration you require.

THE BEAUTY BENEFIT OF EXERCISE

Exercise is hugely beneficial to our skin. It increases blood flow and brings a fresh supply of nutrients to the skin. We breathe more deeply, take in more oxygen, generate happy hormones and also sweat toxins out through the skin. Leading a sedentary lifestyle causes premature ageing, so try to find something that you enjoy that fits easily into your daily routine. You might be able to squeeze in a lunchtime yoga class, do an online workout while the kids are napping or live where there are opportunities to try surfing, riding or climbing.

tip

Commit to a course of classes, as once it's paid for there is more motivation to go along. Some weeks, it won't happen. But be kind to yourself and know that next week will be better.

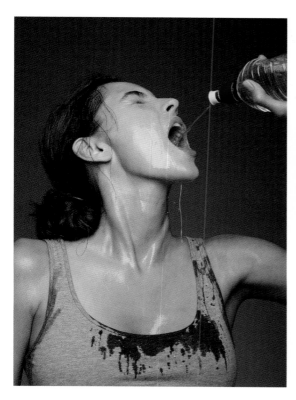
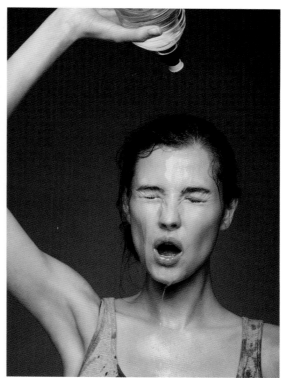
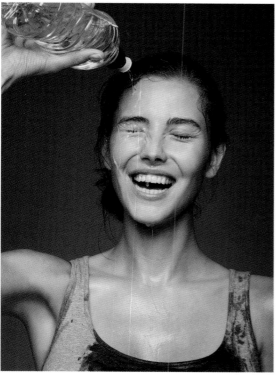
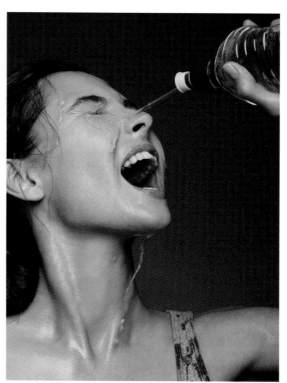

the
TANNING
QUESTION

When exposed to UV rays, our skin seeks to protect itself. Melanocytes are cells that are responsible for creating a pigment called melanin that determines skin tone. The more melanocytes we have, the darker our natural skin colour. When stimulated by the sun, they produce a pigment called melanin that makes our skin adopt that golden glow that we all crave.

I was a child of the eighties, when a deep tan was the main goal of a summer holiday. I fondly remember holidays spent in Spain and France when I'd slather on delicious-smelling oil, then lie out in the sun glistening in a bid to go one shade darker than my friends. Luckily, we now know much more about the links between sun exposure, skin ageing and cancer and are aware of the need to protect our skin by wearing sunscreen.

TOO MUCH SUN – OR NOT ENOUGH?

There are a number of factors to take into consideration. From a health point of view, we need some sun exposure – we are animals and were never intended to live inside or to venture outside only when smothered in sunscreen. We need to allow our skin to absorb some sunlight to enable our bodies to create sufficient vitamin D. Too much, though, can cause at best skin ageing and at worst cancer. UVA rays penetrate the skin to the subcutaneous level, where they can impact on our DNA, compromising the skin's elastin fibres and cause sagging, wrinkles, pigmentation and an uneven surface. They also penetrate glass and clouds, so just because there is cloud cover does not mean you are protected. UVB rays are responsible for both burning (remember 'B' for 'burn') and creating vitamin D.

VITAMIN D

Vitamin D, known as the sunshine vitamin, is not a vitamin in the normal sense, as it's fat-soluble and is made in the body (where it is stored in the liver and kidneys). Without it, the body is unable properly to absorb calcium and our health is at risk from high blood pressure, bowel problems, headaches, restless sleep, low mood, Seasonal Affective Disorder, Parkinson's disease, arthritis, osteoporosis, diabetes, heart disease and cancer. Food sources are scarce. It's mainly found in liver and oily fish (such as tuna, salmon, mackerel and swordfish). There are also small amounts in cheese, milk and mushrooms. Because exposing our skin to UVB rays is the primary means of making vitamin D, we do need to get some sunlight on a daily basis.

The British Skin Foundation recommends that we get 20 minutes of sun exposure a day – without wearing sunscreen – to ensure we have enough vitamin D. The amount we need, however, differs from person to person. It may depend upon your weight, skin type and skin tone. The more melanin you have in your skin and the darker its tone, the more sun exposure you will need to create the same amount of vitamin D. Vitamin D deficiency is more common in women. To ensure you get enough, use a daily sunscreen but maximise your safe full-sun exposure. Also take a daily vitamin D supplement.

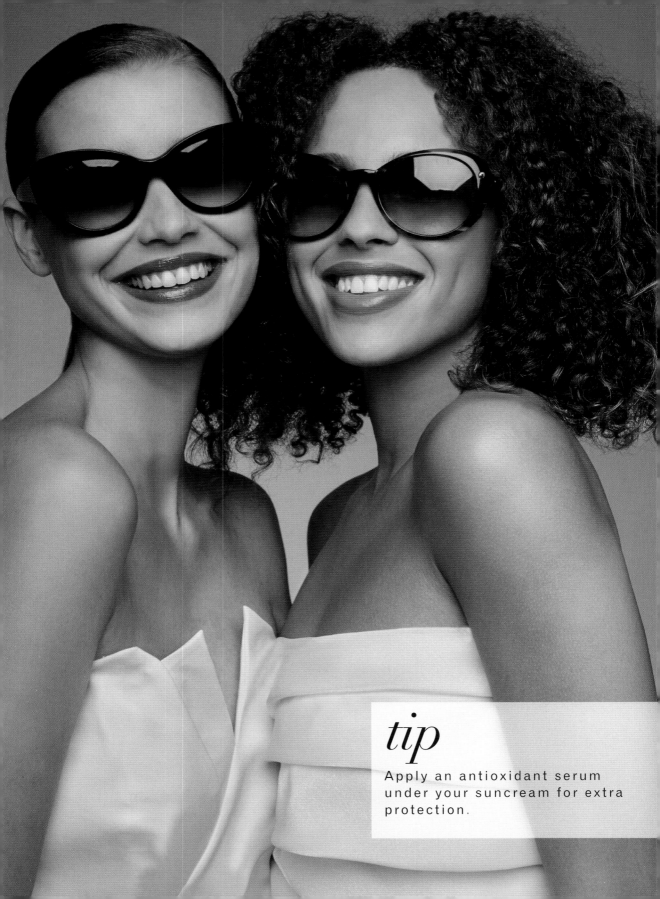

tip

Apply an antioxidant serum under your suncream for extra protection.

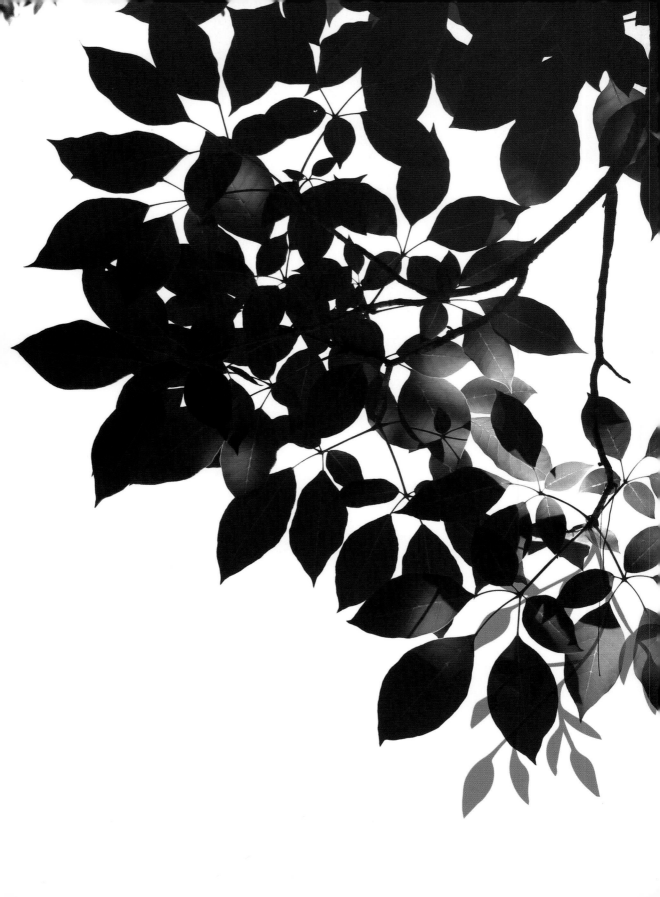

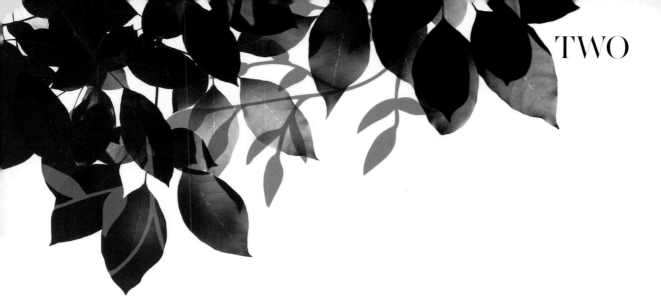

TWO

THE MIND-SKIN CONNECTION

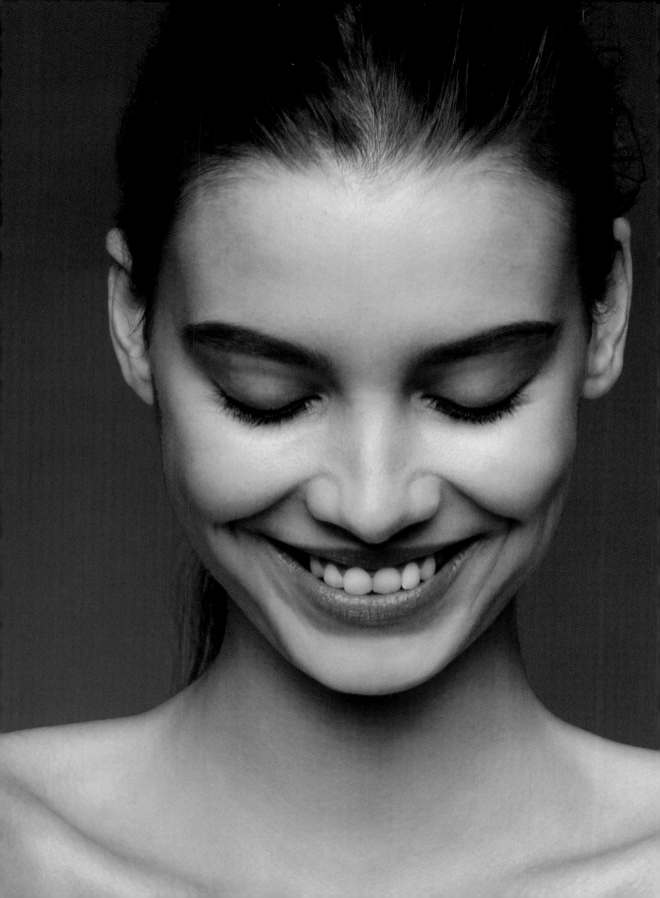

"*Everything* has beauty, but not everyone *sees* it"

CONFUCIUS

the BENEFITS
of MINDFULNESS
and MEDITATION

The skin is our outer protective layer. It takes a battering on our behalf, protecting everything inside the body. Yet it's also our largest sensory organ and an emotional messenger – it's where our hair stands on end when we're frightened, where our blushes confess our embarrassment, the canvas on which we express our sadness when we are upset and our joy when we are happy and where we touch – skin to skin – when we want to show affection. This mind–skin link is what experts call psychodermatology, and it's this science that explains why external skin conditions such as acne, psoriasis, eczema and rosacea are often triggered by internal stress. These visible conditions often dent our self-confidence and, in turn, our stress levels soar even higher. As a result, the mind–skin link becomes an ever more damaging vicious cycle.

Life is 10 per cent of what happens to you and 90 per cent of how you react to it.

Some of the most readily available tools that can help us break this cycle are literally a breath away and cost nothing more than a few moments of our time. Best of all, they're free! Meditation isn't just for the spiritually enlightened. It's a practice that can help all of us live in the moment to become happier and more productive. Countless studies have proven that it can impact positively on both our physical and psychological wellbeing.

You are allowed to be both a masterpiece and a work in progress, simultaneously.

SOPHIA BUSH

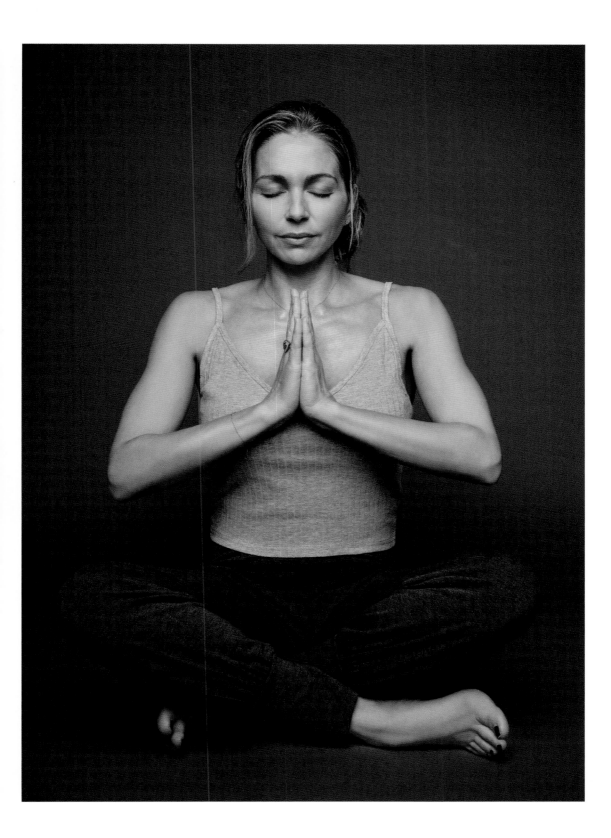

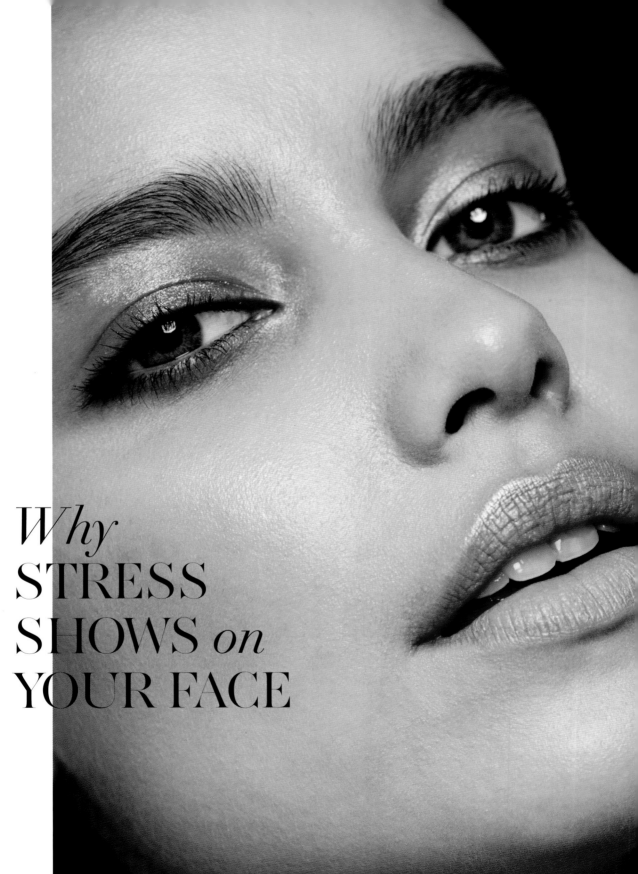

Why
STRESS
SHOWS *on*
YOUR FACE

It's almost impossible to live without some stress in our lives. It's a natural physical response pre-programmed into us to react to a critical situation. When we enter this 'fight or flight' mode, we experience a surge in the hormones adrenalin, cortisol and noradrenalin that prepare us to survive a threat to our lives. Our heart rate accelerates, blood flow to the brain and muscles increases by up to 500 per cent, the conditions inside the stomach become painfully acidic – and even the structure of our collagen and connective tissues is damaged. Although some stress is good for us, triggering our sense of ambition, competitiveness and energy, most of us are living with too much. So it's no wonder we're tense, irritable, anxious and unable to concentrate. The effect of this is cumulative. Over time, it begins to compromise the health of our skin and body. Acne, rosacea, eczema, psoriasis, premature ageing and many other conditions are directly linked to stress levels. Managing these should be a key part of your routine, working alongside any topical products you apply. Remember that stress robs us of sleep – one of the key ingredients we need in order for our skin cells to regenerate overnight.

THE STRESS–SPOT CYCLE

I've seen hundreds of clients with many different skin issues, yet the ones with the most problematic complexions are those living with the most stress. When we're stressed our body releases hormones, which increase oil production in the skin. The result is spots and breakouts, which goes some way to explaining why adult acne is on the rise. Clinical studies indicate that 40 to 55 per cent of the adult population aged twenty to forty have low-grade, persistent acne. According to the *Journal of the American Academy of Dermatology*, 54 per cent of women aged twenty-five and above have some facial acne.

Unfortunately, the stress–skin cycle doesn't stop there. When we eat, the body releases insulin as a means of storing energy for the body.

The more stressed we are, the more insulin we produce. Insulin, in turn, triggers the production of hormones called androgens, which block pores and cause spots. Stress also re-directs blood to the brain and muscles, which is where the body considers it most necessary in order to survive a threatening situation. This is why we talk about blood draining from someone's face when they're frightened or in shock. As blood travels towards the brain and muscles, skin begins to lack the nutrients and oxygen supply it needs to heal these spots.

STRESS AND AGEING

We can tell from someone's expression whether they are happy or stressed. Frowning tightens the facial muscles, which restricts the free flow of blood and nutrients. The more you frown, the more likely it is that worry lines will become permanently ingrained on your face. Stress also triggers a series of chain reactions within the body that accelerate skin ageing:

- *Reduces blood flow*
This means fewer nutrients and less oxygen are being delivered to the skin cells. Over time, this reduces the rate of cell turnover and the skin adopts a pale, lacklustre appearance.

- *Increases cortisol*
When the body produces cortisol, it immediately releases sugars intended to provide the body with energy. Yet not only do these sugars create inflammation within the skin, but cortisol also damages and breaks down the supportive network of collagen and elastin. As the years pass, we develop more lines and wrinkles.

- *Damages DNA*
Small elements called telomeres sit at the ends of DNA strands to stop them from fraying – rather like the ends of shoelaces. Stress 'unravels' these telomeres and if it's a skin cell that's affected, the ageing process rapidly accelerates.

10 TOP TIPS

TO DEAL *with* STRESS

Sadly, a perfectly serene, harmonious life is an unrealistic aim. So, at the very least, if we can't remove it completely, we need to manage our stress better.

These are my *top ten tips*:

1 MEDITATE

Just a few minutes a day can help ease anxiety and stress. I suffered from anxiety at the age of 19 and hypnotherapy taught me the power of a positive mantra. Repeating the words 'cool, calm, collected, confident and courageous' as I meditated helped me to resist the anxiety spirals. Sit up straight with both feet on the floor. Relax your body, close your eyes and take a few deep breaths. Come up with your own positive mantra – anything that resonates with how you want to feel – or just focus on breathing in and out. To start with, set a timer to five minutes; later you can increase this to ten or 15 minutes.

2 BREATHE FROM YOUR BELLY

Breathing from your belly will help you feel calmer, more grounded and more mindful of the present moment, and will also encourage more oxygen to flow around the body, benefiting your complexion. I like to give myself a five-minute break from whatever is bothering me and focus instead on breathing. I follow the pattern 'inhale for the count of five seconds, hold for five, exhale for five'. Make your breath rounded with a smooth flow, so the out breath is just as deep as the in breath. Slowly inhale and exhale through the nose, feeling the breath start in your abdomen and work its way up to the top of your head and back down.

3 WRITE IT DOWN

I often lie awake in bed or wake in the early hours, my head busy with thoughts of all the things I need to do. So I keep a book by my bedside to empty my thoughts on to paper. This helps me drop off to sleep knowing I won't forget anything.

4 LAUGH

You'd be amazed how helpful laughing can be. When we laugh, we release happy hormones, making the body feel relaxed.

5 CUT OUT STIMULANTS

I love a coffee, a glass of wine or some chocolate as much as the next person, but I try always to consume everything in moderation.

6 HAVE A MASSAGE

It eases muscle tension and stimulates nerve endings within the skin to send mental 'relax' messages to the brain. A study at the Touch Research Institute at the University of Miami showed that massage also improved the mood and skin conditions of a group of children suffering from skin redness and itching.

7 TAKE SOME 'ME' TIME

Get outside for a walk, run a warm bath, sit in the park or do a yoga class. Just make sure you put away all digital devices and go somewhere you won't be disturbed.

8 MEET FRIENDS

Friends can help us see things in a different light and make us laugh about a situation that previously felt stressful. Just voicing your anxieties can be therapy in itself.

9 DO ONE HEALTHY THING EACH DAY

Take the stairs at the train station. Swap a piece of fruit or a Beauty Boosting Balls (see page 156) for your usual sweet snack. Switch your morning coffee for a green tea. Change your pasta for brown rice or quinoa. You might find that each beneficial choice keeps you motivated to make healthy decisions in the future.

10 WORK OUT

Physical activity releases endorphins. These reduce our pain receptors and also trigger positive feelings in our body, making us feel happy. Exercise is also an invaluable way of getting rid of pent-up aggression caused by stress.

SLEEPING BEAUTY

It's no secret why we refer to our overnight rest as 'beauty sleep'. When we sleep, our facial muscles fully relax and our body performs the essential functions listed below. When we're sleep-deprived, we develop dark circles under our eyes and find a dull, pallid complexion staring back at us in the mirror. Even one night of lost sleep can have a visible impact.

A study by the University Hospital Case Medical Center in Ohio examined the process of 'catabolysis', or the natural purification process during which skin cells excrete internal waste. The study found that people who got less sleep developed twice the number of premature ageing signs compared to those who managed more shut-eye.

1. PURIFICATION
When we sleep, we perspire, accelerating the body's natural detoxification process, leading to a clearer complexion. Without sleep, the skin becomes clogged, dull and prone to breakouts.

2. REGENERATION
Skin cells renew themselves far more quickly at night than during the day, a process that peaks between 1am and 2am. The production of col-lagen and elastin increases thanks to the peak of growth-hormone secretion at the start of the night. Fewer hours of sleep means slower tissue renewal, leading to a loss of volume and firm-ness and accelerated skin thinning.

3. MICRO-CIRCULATION
Between the hours of 11pm and 4am, while you are asleep, the micro-circulatory system works harder to deliver more oxygen and nutrients to the skin, allowing the cells to regenerate and perform more effectively.

4. MELATONIN PRODUCTION
This hormone, which has antioxidant and anti-inflammatory properties, helps to regulate our sleep/waking rhythm. Peaking at around 2am, it helps to protect skin cells from free-radical damage. When this cycle is thrown out of balance by a lack of sleep, tissue repair is compromised, so the skin becomes more sensitive and susceptible to the visible signs of ageing.

For optimum health we need seven to eight hours of sleep, but achieving this is sometimes easier said than done. I am a long-standing, on/off insomniac, and know there is nothing more frustrating than lying awake in the early hours with a head full of ideas, unable to do something as simple as sleep. These are some tips I have found helpful in restoring my sleep balance.

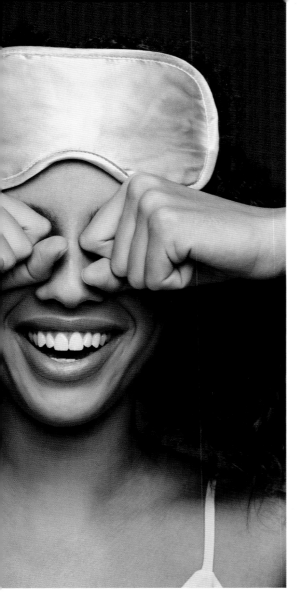
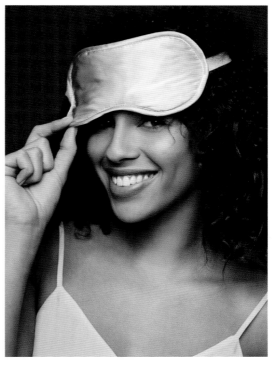
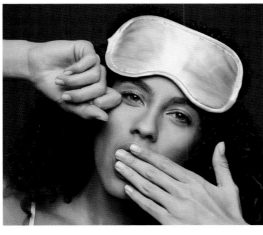
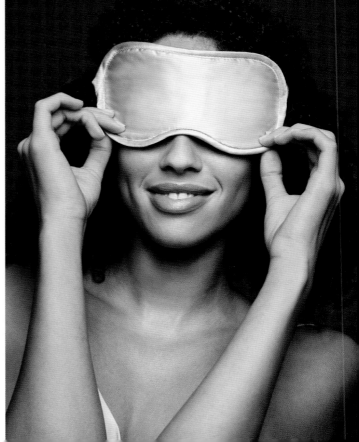

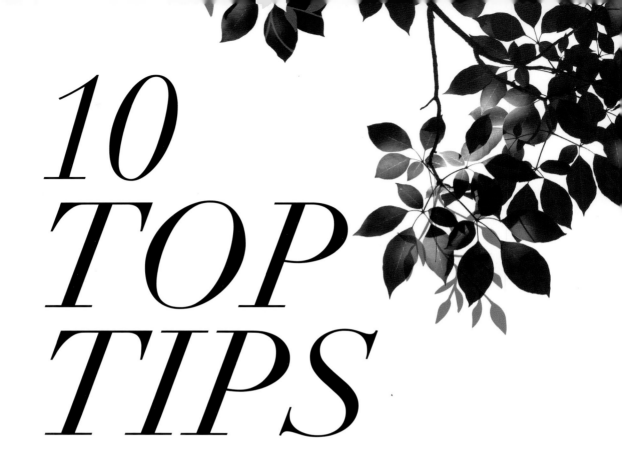

10 TOP TIPS

TO BOOST *your* BEAUTY WHILE *you* SLEEP

For optimum health you need 7–8 hours sleep, but achieving this is sometimes easier said than done. If you have trouble getting the requisite amount, try the following top tips, the first three of which will ensure your skin gets the most benefit.

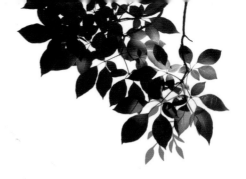

1 CLEANSE

Even if you don't have make-up on, getting rid of pollution, sweat and the grime from the day is vital in order to have vibrant skin.

2 GET OILY

Keep a face oil by the side of your bed and use it to give yourself a five-minute massage. I find massaging acupressure points really helpful; not only does it nourish the skin overnight, it also helps relax the mind.

3 SLEEP ON YOUR BACK

It helps to prevent wrinkles! If we sleep on our sides, our faces get compressed into our pillows. When this is repeated night after night, it causes short-term creases to develop into permanent lines.

4 WEAR A MASK

I have been doing this for years. An eye mask not only supports the delicate skin around the eyes but the secure feeling it gives is comforting. The darkness it creates tells the brain that the sun has gone, it's now time for our natural body clock to slow down and switch off.

5 CREATE A BEDTIME ROUTINE

Go for a gentle walk outside or do five minutes of yin yoga or meditation to help your mind switch off. Instead of counting sheep, try counting backwards in threes from 300. I very rarely get past 260!

6 AVOID ALL SCREENS

The blue light given off by computers, phones and televisions sends signals to the brain that it's time to wake up.

7 CREATE A BALANCE IN YOUR BODY TEMPERATURE

Overheating can keep your body awake, so sleep with a window open. Have a thin cotton sheet under your duvet so you have different layers you can throw off throughout the night. Keep a damp flannel by the side of your bed or a water spritz to cool yourself. Bed socks may not be sexy but if your feet are warm the rest of your body will feel warm.

8 DRINK A HERBAL TEA

Chamomile has a calming effect on the central nervous system – my children love this with a teaspoon of honey – or a sleep tea blend with hops and valerian, which is perfect for telling the body it's time to switch off.

9 USE SOME AROMATHERAPY OILS

Massage lavender, chamomile, valerian or marjoram oil behind your ears or on to your pulse points to induce a calming sensation within the body. Or simply sprinkle a few drops on your pillow.

10 HAVE A BEDTIME SNACK

Snacking on Brazil nuts or walnuts just before you go to bed can have a beneficial effect. Both contain protein, potassium and selenium – all of which help boost production of the 'sleep hormone' melatonin. My children and I also like to snack on bananas as they contain potassium and magnesium, which relax muscular tension. Bananas are also rich in an amino acid called tryptophan, which is converted to serotonin, a hormone that helps us drift off to sleep easily.

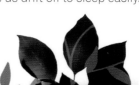

THE POWER
of YOGA

Yoga is like a management system for modern-day stress and is beneficial for both the mind and the body in a number of ways:

When I first encountered yoga I found its slow pace maddening. As a young, energetic 19-year-old I preferred to spend my time in more intense gym classes – if I wasn't working up a sweat, I didn't feel like I was working out. Eight years later, faced with the demands of juggling work with bringing up a young family, I attended a class in central London. Suddenly, it was a like a light bulb had been switched on! I left feeling calm and uplifted for the first time in ages. These days, yoga has become an essential part of my life.

- ### PHYSICAL STRENGTH
Yoga is all about using your natural body weight to build strength without developing bulky muscles. It works to create the long, lean muscle we crave – as well as increasing stamina and improving posture.

- ### JOINT HEALTH & FLEXIBILITY
We were not made to lead a sedentary lifestyle, yet many of us spend each day sitting at a computer. Yoga encourages us to enhance our natural joint movement and flexibility, keeping us supple as we age. Many athletes incorporate yoga into their training regimen, and it can be a great way to prevent arthritis.

- ### BREATHING
Many of us take short, shallow breaths from our chest – rather than long, deep ones from our stomach. The result is a reduced supply of oxygen and nutrients being delivered to the organs. Shallow breathing also makes us more susceptible to panic attacks. Pranayama is a yogic breathing technique that encourages deep, slow, rhythmic breathing, which calms the mind and body – and nourishes the skin.

- ### BLOOD FLOW
The movements of yoga increase blood flow through muscles and tissues, delivering a fresh supply of oxygen and nutrients to cells and keeping organs – including the skin – healthy.

- ### IMMUNITY & DETOXIFICATION
The relaxation and breathing techniques of a yogic practice send a calming message to the immune and nervous systems. The rhythmic, flowing movements also enhance the flow of the lymphatic system, the body's defence mechanism that keeps our internal fluids in balance and aids our natural detoxification process.

- ### HAPPINESS
During a yoga practice there's so much to focus on in terms of your breath, posture and the position you're trying to hold, that there's little opportunity to fret about your regular worries. It's amazing how much clearer your mind feels when you emerge.

- ### HORMONES
When we get stressed, the glands of the endocrine system secrete the hormone cortisol into the body. Yoga has a calming, rejuvenating effect on these glands, reducing stress and the damaging effects it has on the skin.

Here are some of my favourite yoga poses for vibrant skin. Practise them individually, holding each one for up to a minute. Or combine them into a complete yoga flow. A word of caution: those with high or low blood pressure, neck or back injuries and pregnant women should consult their doctor before attempting any exercise.

▶ STANDING FORWARD BEND
(Uttanasana)

1. A simple posture that increases blood flow to the head. I often do it while the kettle is boiling first thing in the morning.

2. Stand with your legs hip distance apart. Raise your hands above your head. Breathe in and bend slightly backwards.

3. Bend forwards from the hips, breathing out as you do. Bring your hands down to the floor just in front of you, bending your knees if you need to. An alternative I love because it adds extra weight to the fold is to cross your forearms and hold your elbows in a rag doll pose.

4. To take this pose one step further progress to a wide leg forward bend (see page 44).

Yoga can be a vital element in effective skincare as its positive impact on the mind and body carries added benefits for our complexions.

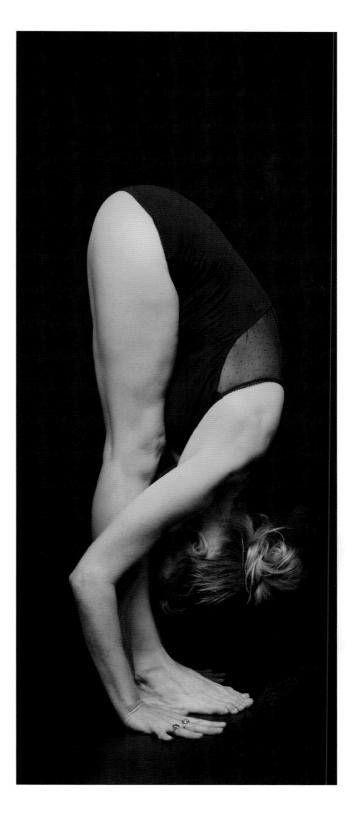

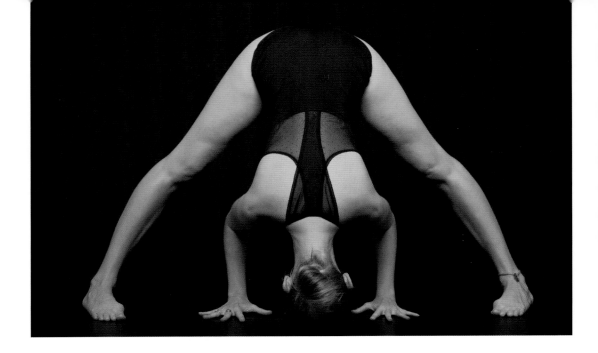

Yoga reduces stress and the harmful effects it has on skin

▲ PRASARITA PADOTTANASANA

1. Stand with your legs further than hip width apart but not uncomfortably wide. Place your hands on your hips, lift your torso up and bend forward, placing your palms on the floor in front of you. Relax and hold for five breaths.

2. To release the pose, place your hands on your hips and slowly roll up through the spine to a standing position.

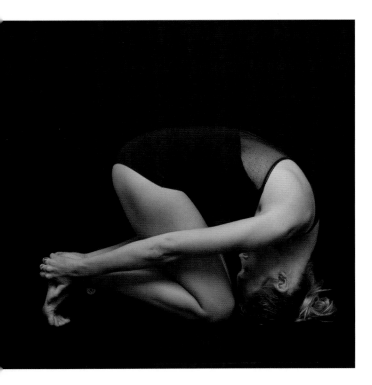

◀ RABBIT POSE *(Shashankasana)*

This pose relaxes the mind, increases blood flow to the head, relieves tension in the upper back and allows nutrients to flow towards the face.

1. From child's pose, take your arms to your sides and reach for your heels.

2. Inhale as you slowly roll forward until the crown of your head is on the floor, with your hips lifted directly above your knees.

3. Tuck your chin in towards your chest and hold for 30 seconds, breathing slowly.

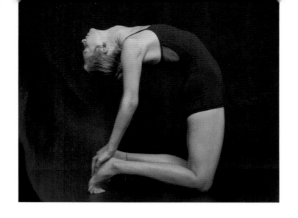

> Yoga supports the lymphatic system, the body's natural detoxification process, making for clearer, more vibrant skin.

▼ COBRA POSE *(Bhujangasana)*

Opens up the chest, allowing extra oxygen to flow into the body. It also aids the removal of toxins, supporting the liver for clearer skin.

1. Lie on your stomach with your legs straight, feet together and your forehead on the floor.

2. Place your hands by your shoulders and keep your elbows close to your body.

3. Push up, lifting your head, chest and stomach off the floor as you exhale (keeping the belly button on the floor).

4. Inhale and gently arch your back and straighten your arms as you tilt your chin upwards.

5. Gently lower your body back down to the floor as you exhale.

▲ CAMEL POSE *(Ustrasana)*

This pose is an intense backbend that opens up the chest, increasing lung capacity and allowing more oxygen to flow through the body.

1. Kneel on the floor with your knees hip distance apart.

2. Reach your hands back one at a time to grasp your heels.

3. Allow your hips to press forwards as your shoulder blades move inwards and downwards.

4. Gently arch your head back, opening your throat while keeping your buttocks and belly soft.

5. Rotate your arms so that the elbow creases face outwards as you breathe gently. Hold for 30 to 60 seconds.

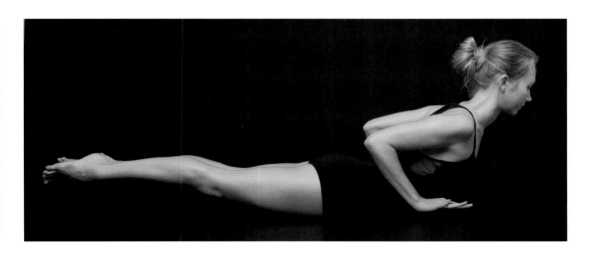

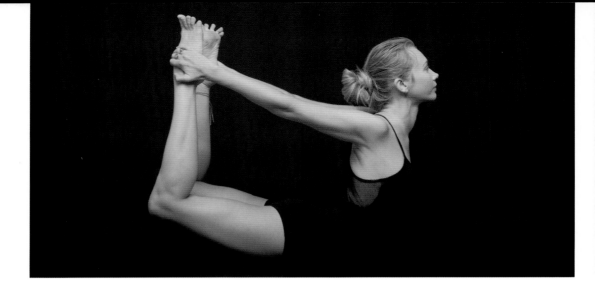

> As a form of exercise, yoga increases heart rate and blood flow, so the skin receives a greater supply of oxygen and nutrients.

▲ **BOW POSE** *(Dhanurasana)*
Supports the digestion and overall health.

1. Lie on your stomach with your hands by your sides. Bend your knees up so that your heels are close to your buttocks.

2. Arch your back slightly until you can take hold of your ankles with both hands.

3. Using strength from both your legs and arms, try to pull your ankles closer towards your head as you rock forwards and backwards on your stomach.

◀ **LION POSE** *(Simhasana)*
A great stress reliever. It relaxes facial tension and increases happiness!

1. Sit on your mat cross-legged with your hands gently resting on your knees.

2. Breathe in deeply through your nose and squeeze your eyes tightly closed. As you do so, clench all of the muscles in your face, and make tight fists with your hands.

3. Exhale fast as you open your eyes and mouth wide, stick out your tongue, unclench your fists and stretch your fingers. Hold for five seconds.

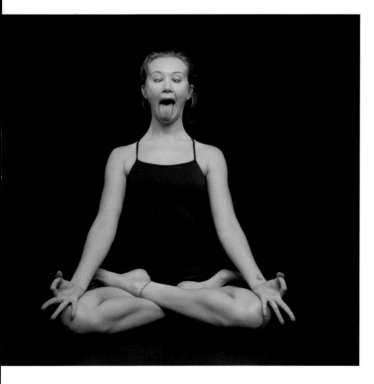

▶ SHOULDER STAND
(Salamba Sarvangasana)

Reverses the effects of gravity. Inversions bring blood to the head and are one of the best ways to enhance facial radiance.

1. Lie on your back with your arms by your side, your palms facing down.

2. Lift your legs up, raising the hips up off the floor as you do so.

3. Supporting your lower back with your hands, roll up on to your shoulders and find your balance. Hold for as long as you like.

You can extend this into:

▼ PLOUGH POSE *(Halasana)*

1. Supporting your lower back with your hands, slowly continue to move your legs over your head at a 180-degree angle, until your toes touch the floor behind your head.

2. Relax into the pose and hold for a minute.

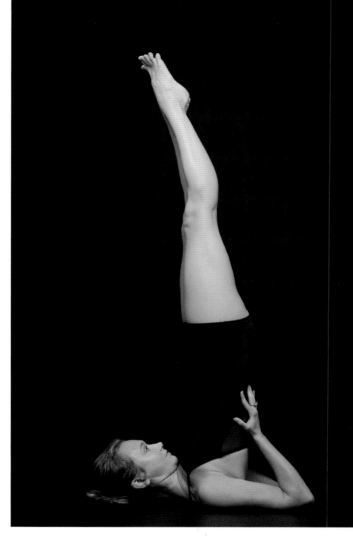

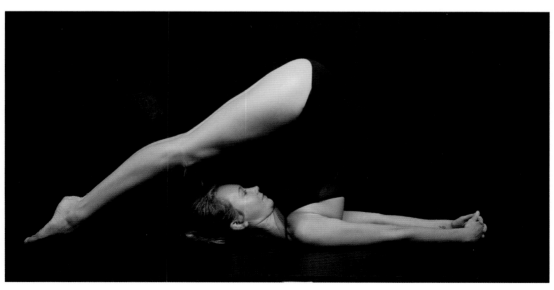

Yoga creates a positive feedback loop. Beginning or ending the day in a healthy, mindful way encourages you to make further positive choices.

▼ FISH POSE *(Matsyasana)*

Tones the muscles of your face and throat. It also supports the hormonal system, the thyroid, pineal and pituitary glands. A great way to help combat hormonal breakouts.

1. Lie on your back with your legs straight, your feet together and your arms by your sides.

2. Place your hands underneath your hips, palms facing down. Bring the elbows closer towards each other beneath your body.

3. Breathe in as you raise your head and chest up. Keeping the chest elevated, lower your head backwards until you can rest the crown of your head on the floor.

4. Keep the neck arched and your chin lifted up to the ceiling as you press your thighs into the floor. Hold the pose for as long as you can.

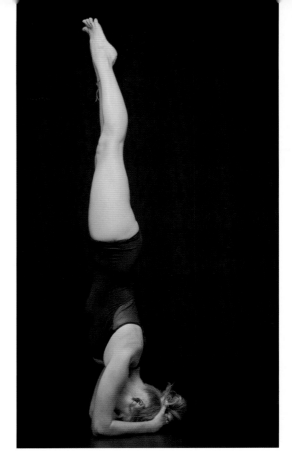

▲ HEAD STAND

My ultimate skin and head benefiting pose – it really increases blood flow and allows you to totally switch off.

1. Kneel on the floor, interlace your fingers together and place your forearms on the floor with elbows out wide. Place the crown of your head in the space created between your arms with your head closely up against your hands.

2. Half pose – keep your tiptoes on the floor, lift your knees up so your legs are straight and raise your hips to create an inverted 'V' shape. Breathe deeply. Hold this for as long as is comfortable.

3. Full pose – walk your feet closer to your body. Lift both feet up away from the floor at the same time and continue to lift the legs straight up into the air. Hold for as long as you can.

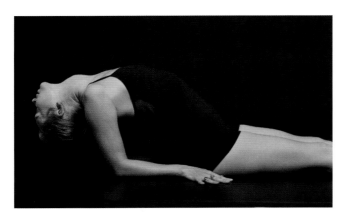

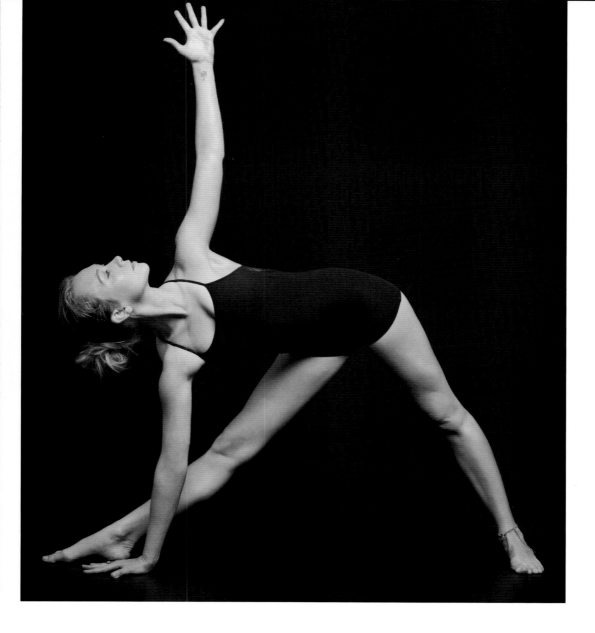

▲ TRIANGLE POSE (*Trikonasana*)

This is about balancing the mind and body, opening the chest and heart, increasing oxygen to the head and whole body, refreshing and reviving the complexion. A good stress reliever that stimulates internal organs.

1. Stand with your feet just more than hip width apart.

2. Turn your right foot out pointing forwards and left foot in by about 15 degrees.

3. Keeping the pelvis facing forwards, take a deep breath, as you exhale, bend your body downwards to the right, taking your right arm straight down towards the floor and resting it on your ankle or on the floor. Stretch your left arm straight up in the air. Rotate your head to gaze up at your palm.

4. Relax and breathe into the pose. Reverse the pose and repeat to the other side.

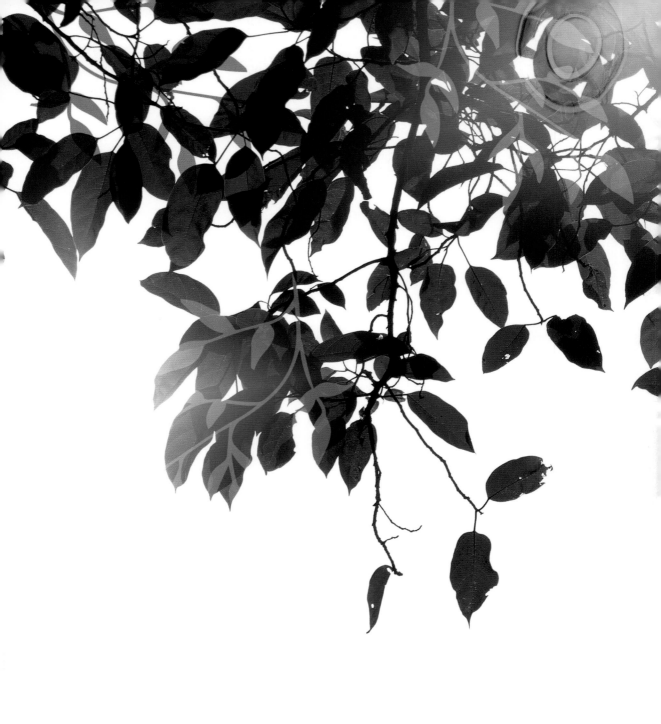

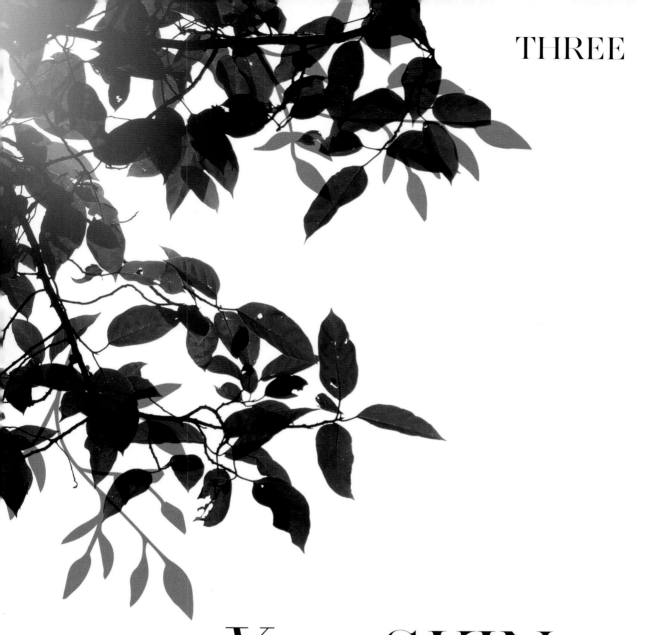

THREE

Your SKIN THROUGH THE AGES

Your TEENS

Not all teens will experience skin issues. There's often a connection between genetics and how your skin will fare – the fact is that we can't fight the internal hormones doing what mother nature intended – but the great news is that there are ways to support the skin, no matter what might be happening on and beneath the surface.

Focus: balance oil production & maintain skin health

If your skin is playing up, it's likely to be because your levels of testosterone have risen. This increases sebum production and makes the skin oilier. At the same time, keratin (one of the main skin-building blocks) becomes more abundant. Increased amounts of both sebum and keratin blocks pores, which encourages bacteria and spots to form. In some cases, the skin becomes inflamed and spots develop into acne. If your concern is sensitivity, it might be that you've started using the wrong skincare products. Too harsh, too synthetic or highly perfumed products may have this effect. Alternatively, it could be that your skin is naturally dry and needs a gentler approach.

SKIN CHANGES
- Sebaceous glands get bigger
- Oil production increases
- More keratin is produced, making the skin thicker
- A weak skin barrier, resulting in spots or sensitivity
- Cell turnover is around 28 days

COMMON PROBLEMS
- Spots
- Sensitivity
- Blackheads
- Shine and excess oil

THE REALITY
You may have chosen to go on to birth control, which also disrupts your natural hormone balance. Exam stress is another factor.

CHOOSING THE RIGHT PRODUCTS
Unfortunately, there isn't a magic potion to bust spots in seconds. Traditional treatments can be harsh, leaving the skin feeling clean but stripping it of its natural oils, which the skin strives to replace by overproducing a fresh supply. This is what brings on that midday shine. The key to breaking the cycle is effective cleansing. Opt for a gentle gel wash morning and night over the entire face, then apply a targeted treatment product directly to the spot. These usually contain salicylic acid, which has antibacterial properties. Natural alternatives

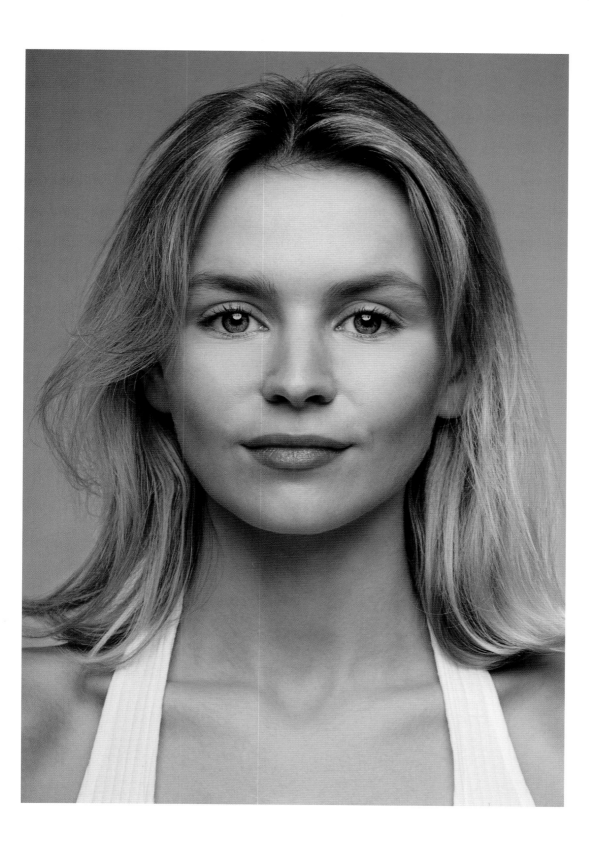

are tea tree oil and essential oils such as lavender. Use at night and wash off in the morning, as most essential oils make the skin more sensitive to sunlight. Before bedtime, apply a small amount of dry oil. Once a week, use a balancing or deep-cleansing face mask – aloe vera, clay, salicylic acid, mud and honey.

TIME FOR A PROFESSIONAL TREATMENT?

These are usually unnecessary, but if your skin is becoming spottier or blackheads bug you, a deep-cleansing facial or a course of LED light therapy will help.

LISTEN TO YOUR SKIN

We've all had it drummed into us that we should be using a moisturiser every single day, but if it's merely making yours greasier, then try applying it every other day and see how your complexion responds. If you're using a spot-busting product containing salicylic acid, make sure you give it time to work – usually a skin cycle of a month – and be sure to balance it with a hydrating oil or serum, as it will dry the skin.

diet

CUT DOWN ON

- Cow's milk.
- Sugar – if you crave fizzy drinks, try kombucha (a fermented, naturally fizzy drink, traditionally made from sweetened black or white tea, and packed with good gut bacteria) or sparkling water with cranberry juice and a teaspoon of honey.

EAT MORE OF

- Zinc, as it balances hormones.
- Seeds such as sesame, flaxseed, sunflower and pumpkin. They contain zinc, magnesium and essential fatty acids, which are vital for skin function.

KEY FOODS TO EAT

- Bananas.
- Pumpkin seeds.
- Broccoli.
- Milk alternatives such as coconut, hemp, almond.

Do...

CLEANSE daily, morning and night

KEEP IT SIMPLE – sometimes less is more

APPLY a tiny amount of an oil at night to rebalance sebum levels

DO APPLY a weekly mask

DRINK water

Don't...

USE products containing mineral oils, such as petroleum oil. These block pores and make the skin look dehydrated and dull

OVER-STRIP THE SKIN – it's not 'dirty', it's simply out of balance

USE NIGHT CREAMS as they're too heavy for young skin

OVER-EXFOLIATE as it can lead to sensitivity – once a week is a good starting point

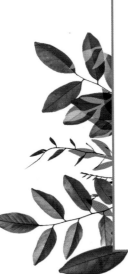

Your
TWENTIES

Focus: balance oil production, maintain skin health and protect it from future damage.

The hardest period in life is one's 20s. It's a shame because you're your most gorgeous, and you're physically in peak condition. But it's actually when you're most insecure and full of self-doubt. When you don't know what's going to happen, it's frightening.'

HELEN MIRREN

Unless you're battling acne, the chances are that you can get away with a minimal skincare routine at this age. This is a time in your life when your skin is in its prime as cell turnover is still optimal. 'Protection and prevention' should be your mantra. From the age of twenty-five our collagen production begins to decline but you won't see the visible signs on your skin yet.

By the time you reach your late twenties, you may start to notice your first signs of ageing. This could be fine lines around the eyes as skin here is thinner and more delicate than on the rest of the face. If you've been a sun worshiper or a smoker, both factors will drastically accelerate the rate at which your skin ages.

SKIN CHANGES
- Spots still occur
- Collagen production begins to slow
- Pores become visibly larger
- Skin cell turnover decelerates

COMMON PROBLEMS
- Spots
- Excessive shine
- Sensitivity due to inflammation caused by overly harsh skincare or acne medicated creams
- Blackheads
- Scarring and pitting from acne
- Fine lines beginning to show
- Combination skin – dry with spots

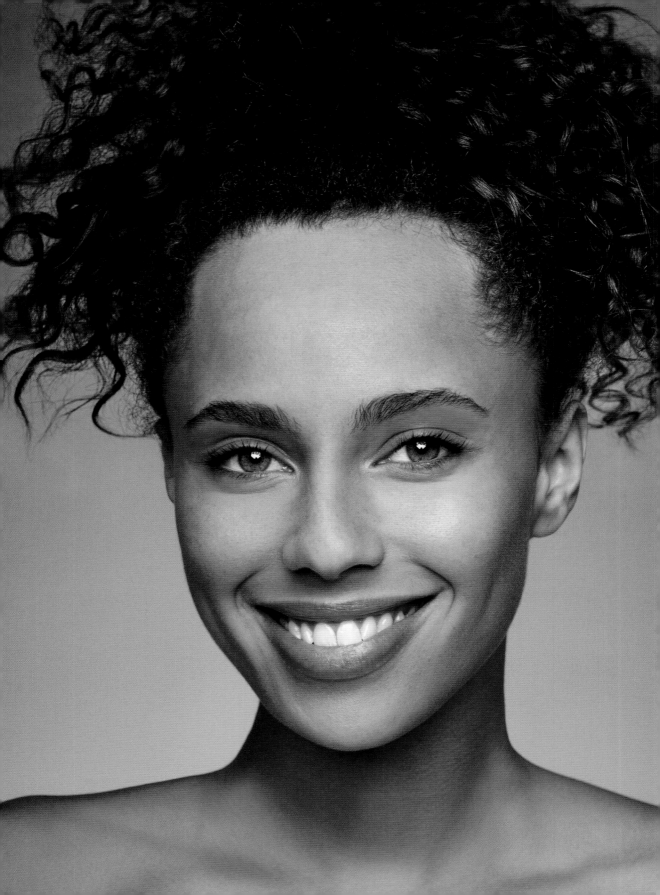

THE REALITY

You're likely to be burning the candle at both ends. You feel invincible and would rather have a golden tan than bother with a skincare routine! You might be sleeping in your make-up and not have the budget for facials or expensive products. This is a period of transition, when you move from the pressures of school to the stress of university or working life – probably in a new city where pollution levels are higher. It's easy to develop bad habits. You grab a latte on the way to work, skip lunch and reach for the sugary snacks when the mid-afternoon slump hits. You have no time for the scheduled sports you did at school and may be on the contraceptive pill, which disrupts your hormones. Psychologically, this is the age when we can become most critical of ourselves. The late nights, sun bathing and sugar overload might not show on your face during this decade, but they will do so in your next one.

CHOOSING THE RIGHT PRODUCTS

Think quick and affordable. Cleanse morning and evening with a gel-based cleanser if you have oily or combination skin, or use a cream-based cleanser if you're prone to dryness or sensitivity. Moisturise every morning, picking lighter textures as a general rule. You don't need a heavy anti-wrinkle cream at this age. Exfoliating twice a week will brighten and refresh your skin. The biggest weapon in your skin protection armoury is sunscreen – so wear it every day! Apply a home face mask once every two weeks to keep your skin looking nourished and vibrant.

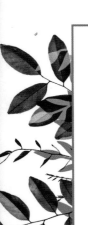
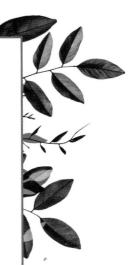

Do...

Get into a DAILY skincare routine

WEAR an SPF daily, all year round

Don't...

SMOKE – it interferes with blood flow, limiting the amount of oxygen and nutrients that reach the skin. The action of drawing on a cigarette alone will cause you to develop lines around your mouth

HAVE BOTOX – you seriously don't need it!

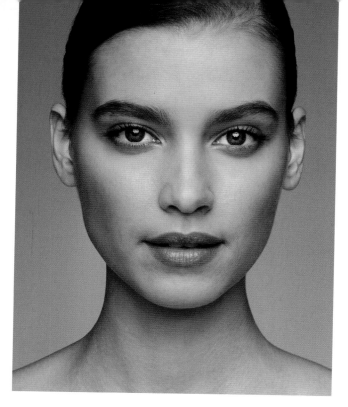

diet

What we eat affects the condition of our skin at every age and a few small tweaks now can make a big difference to how your skin ages.

CUT DOWN ON

- Sugar and stimulants (such as coffee), as these fuel hormones in the body.

EAT MORE OF

- Foods rich in vitamin C such as peppers, watercress, cabbage, broccoli, cauliflower, strawberries, lemons, kiwi fruit, peas, melons, oranges, limes and tomatoes.

- Essential fatty acids that help balance hormones. Find these in flax and chia seeds, oils or supplements (evening primrose oil, borage, coconut or flax oil), avocado, raw nuts and cold-water fish.

TIME FOR A PROFESSIONAL TREATMENT?

If you haven't experienced a facial yet, now is a good time to start. Choose a treatment with a facialist or a brand you like. Facial massage is great for lowering stress levels. A deep cleanse, LED and high-frequency and galvanic treatments are also things to look out for. If you're getting spots, look for a gentle enzyme peel to rebalance your skin.

LISTEN TO YOUR SKIN

Using a heavy anti-ageing cream will most likely bring you out in spots. Prevention is better than cure at this age. If your skin is dry but has spots, you need two types of cleanser: a cream or milk to remove make-up on a daily basis, and a gel wash with antibacterial properties to treat spots. If you were to use this wash morning and night, it would be too drying for your skin.

If you are developing spots, don't use your moisturiser at night. Imagine a tiny grain of rice and use this amount only of an oil to help rebalance your skin without clogging the pores.

DO IT NOW!

Sleep! Schedule some catch-up nights. Think of sleep as being part of your skincare routine – it's a time for your complexion to rebalance and repair itself.

Develop some stress management skills. Your job will still be there in the morning! Taking some time out will make you more productive and help manage stress levels.

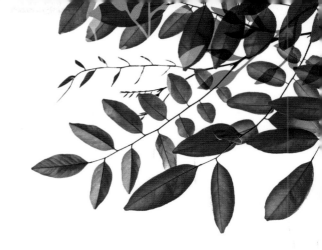

Your THIRTIES

Focus: correct & protect

Beauty is how you feel inside, and it reflects in your eyes. It is not something physical.'

SOPHIA LOREN

It is now that life factors such as pregnancy and motherhood may affect your skin. Collagen production slows down by around 1 per cent each year at this point, so you'll start to see the physical signs of ageing appear around your eyes and on your forehead. Despite this, this decade is often the time when you begin to feel more confident and comfortable in your own skin. With the correct care, your skin can really glow during this decade!

SKIN CHANGES
- Collagen and elastin fibres become less effective
- Cell renewal continues to slow and skin can become thicker
- Glycation may start to become visible
- Fine lines around the eye area will start to deepen

COMMON PROBLEMS
- Dark circles
- More visible lines
- Sensitivity heightened in the form of flushing, reactive skin
- Melasma and hormone-related pigmentation
- Acne

THE REALITY
You might be dating, planning a wedding, a pregnancy, building an empire, on and off birth control, travelling. This is the age of multitasking! And yes, you may still be experiencing spots, but now with the added visibility of the ageing process.

CHOOSING THE RIGHT PRODUCTS

Your mantra here is 'protection, prevention and reverse'. This means cleansing, applying a serum and following it with an SPF. Now is also the time to add in an eye cream. Cell turnover is slowing and the skin is thickening, so exfoliating once a week will help keep the skin looking fresh and allow your serums to be absorbed more easily. Key ingredients to look out for include antioxidants (especially vitamin C) and retinol.

TIME FOR A PROFESSIONAL TREATMENT?

Even if you don't have any specific skin concerns, getting into the routine of having a facial every eight weeks is generally a good idea. Some good options are microcurrent, oxygen, LED light, microdermabrasion, facial massage, facial reflexology and gentle peels.

diet

What we eat can affect the condition of our skin at every age and a few small tweaks can make a big difference.

EAT MORE OF

- Vitamin C-rich foods play a huge role in collagen production. So enjoy plenty of raw peppers, citrus fruits, broccoli and leafy greens.

- Antioxidants prevent the impact of oxidative stress on your skin and in turn, forestall premature ageing. Find them in red, orange and yellow vegetables, leafy greens, onion and garlic, raw fruits, seeds, nuts and their oils plus basil.

Do...

MAKE FACIALS part of your regular routine. Once every two to three months is a good starting point

ADD SERUMS into your home skincare routine

Don't...

SLEEP with your make-up on

Even if you don't have any specific skin concerns, getting into the routine of having a facial every eight weeks is generally a good idea.

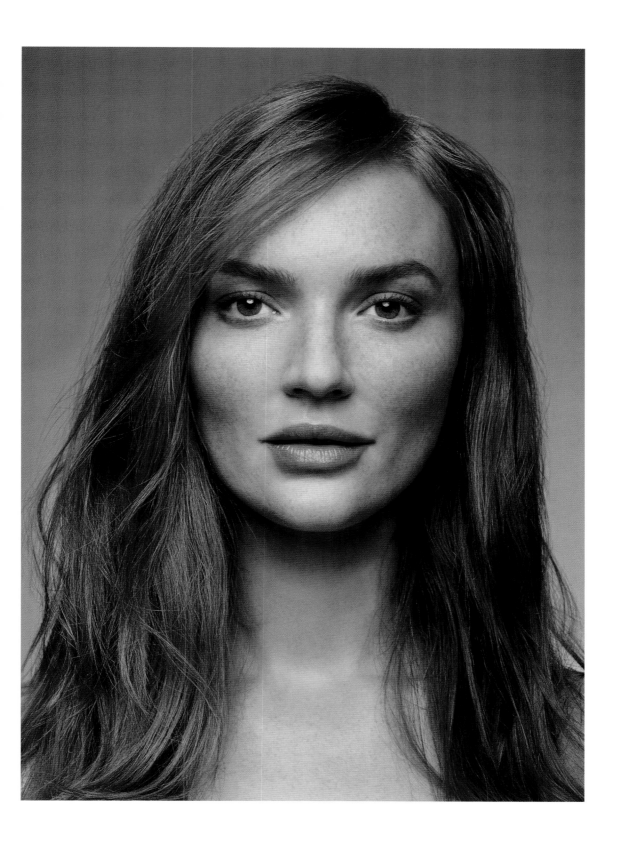

Your FERTILE YEARS & PREGNANCY

As hormones have such a huge impact on how our skin looks and feels, both contraception and being pregnant can really affect our complexion.

THE CONTRACEPTIVE PILL

I've seen clients in their twenties and thirties who suffer from breakouts and acne on a regular basis as a result of being on or off the pill. There are a number of different pills available, with different levels of synthetic hormones. In some cases, the pill is actually used to help prevent acne. The combined pill increases oestrogen, which can result in oestrogen dominance. The reason it is often prescribed for acne is that the higher levels of oestrogen mask the male androgen hormones that are often the culprits of acne. But, this doesn't treat the root cause, and once you come off the pill, it will most likely return. The progesterone-only pill doesn't create oestrogen dominance, but can cause breakouts. There is also a connection between the pill and the development of melasma.

POLYCYSTIC OVARY DISORDER (PCOS)

You may be experiencing acne and not able to discover the root cause. In such cases, I always suggest that clients visit their GP or gynaecologist to rule out PCOS as a possibility. Lifestyle and diet are a key factor in managing this condition and both your home skincare regimen and professional treatments can help.

IVF

The lead-up, actual treatment and after-effects of assisted reproduction can be physically challenging, not to mention highly emotional. We've already seen how stress affects the body and skin. The specific skin issues associated with assisted reproduction can vary quite widely – from acne to extreme dryness and sensitivity. During this time, the ideal is to keep your skincare simple, avoiding highly perfumed and synthetic ingredients and retinols.

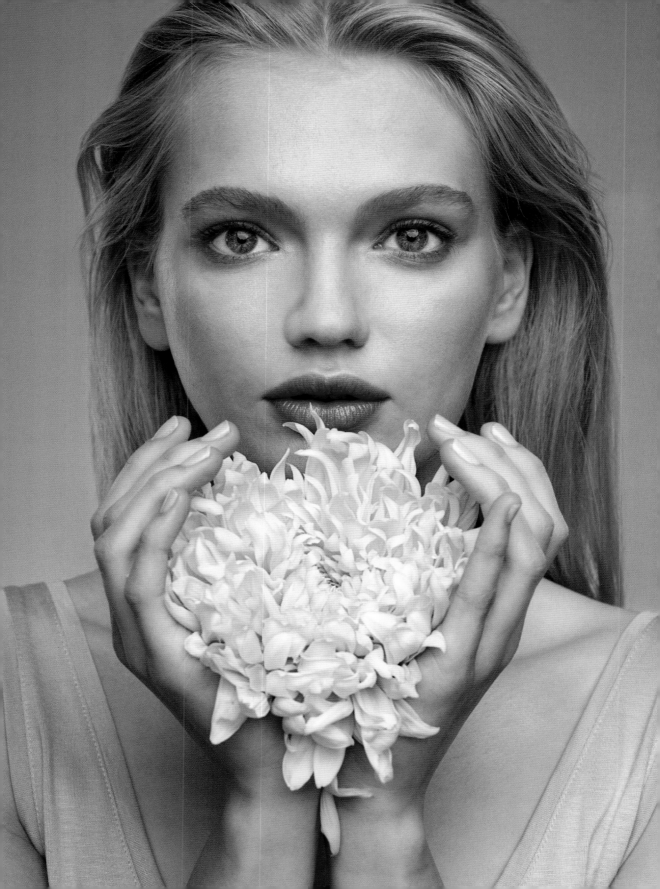

Pregnancy

Although some women breeze through pregnancy, enjoying a 'pregnancy glow', others' experience is quite the opposite. About 70 per cent develop melasma or chloasma – dark spots on the face and arms known as the 'mask of pregnancy'. This disappears in the months following birth. Your acne and eczema may get worse while pregnant, while psoriasis may improve.

Changes to your skin
- Progesterone can increase as much as 60 per cent, which increases the amount of fat stored by the body.
- Oestrogen can increase by as much as 30 per cent.
- The volume of blood can almost double, which explains the 'healthy glow'.

Chloasma/melasma
This occurs as a result of an increase in the pigment-stimulating hormones during pregnancy. It develops as patches on the cheeks, upper lip, chin and forehead and is often genetic (more than 30 per cent of people will have a family history of melasma). The second contributing factor is sun exposure. It fades after pregnancy but can reoccur if you have repeated or extensive sun exposure or if you become pregnant again. The best solution is to wear a high SPF on a daily basis.

Pregnancy breakouts
With hormones in abundance and anxiety levels high, skin can respond with hormonal breakouts, especially around the chin and jawline.

Extreme sensitivity/rosacea
Skin can become more sensitive during pregnancy, particularly to certain products, temperature and sun exposure. It's thought that this is our body's way of protecting itself and the foetus from infection and disease. It also explains why we go off certain smells and foods that we previously enjoyed. As blood volume increases, it's no wonder we feel like we have an internal radiator!

Product ingredients to avoid
If your skincare products contain any of the following you should seek medical advice before using them:
- **Vitamin A/retinol** – they speed up cell turnover but also make the skin much more prone to sun damage and developing pigmentation. There have also been studies that link retinol-based products and birth/child defects, so continue to avoid vitamin A products whilst breastfeeding.
- **Phthalates/formaldehyde/toluene** – these chemicals are often found in perfume and nail polishes. Research is being carried out to assess a possible link with birth defects.
- **Ammonia** – often found in hair dyes, it has carcinogenic properties, so steer clear.
- **Dihydroxyacetone** – found in self-tanning products. Inhalation can be harmful to both mother and foetus.

Your essential pregnancy skincare routine

- Cleanse twice daily before applying a serum and moisturiser.

- Gentle exfoliation weekly.

- High SPF daily.

- Mask once weekly for a specific skin issue, such as calming, sensitivity, flushing or breakouts.

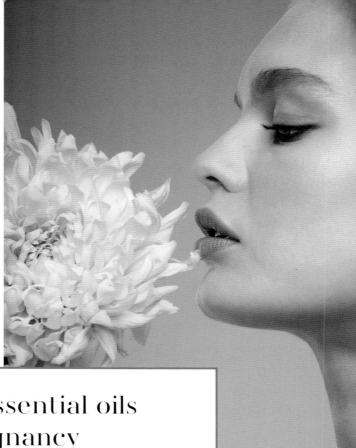

a guide to essential oils in pregnancy

AVOID

Basil – encourages menstruation.

Chamomile blue – encourages menstruation.

Cypress – acts as a diuretic and has a regulating effect on the menstrual cycle.

Jasmine – can stimulate uterine contractions.

Juniper berry – it's a diuretic.

Rosemary – it's highly stimulating.

USE

Frankincense – it's uplifting and deepens breathing.

Geranium – hormone balancing, good for stress-related conditions. A sedative, yet uplifting to the nervous system.

Ginger – amazing for combating nausea.

Mandarin – great for relieving stress and nervous tension. Also excellent for treating stretch marks when mixed with a carrier plant oil.

Neroli – a sedative, good for anxiety and depression.

Your FORTIES

At this age, oestrogen, which keeps our skin hydrated and plump while maintaining cell turnover, begins to decline and the body becomes more vulnerable to the effects of testosterone.

Focus: re-energise, repair, firm & protect the skin.

Your face is marked with lines of life, put there by love and laughter, suffering and tears. It's beautiful.

LYNSAY SANDS

You will be able to see the visible signs of ageing as your skin develops fine lines and sun spots and begins to lose firmness. It may also look dull and lack the vibrancy it once had. Much like in our teens, in our forties we can experience breakouts, though the skin can become drier with a more dull appearance. Unwanted facial hair is another undesirable side effect.

SKIN CHANGES
- Continued slowdown of cell renewal within the epidermal layer
- Reduced fibroblast activity, muscle tone slackens
- Reduced spring-ability of elastin fibres
- Reduced skin density of collagen fibres
- Possible overactive, pressured capillary network resulting in thread veins
- Increased sebum production and some hormonal spots
- Reduction of hyaluronic acid within the skin making it feel drier

COMMON PROBLEMS
- Ageing around the eyes
- Deepening expression lines
- Pigmentation patches
- Eyelids slacken, fold lines at the sides of the mouth become more noticeable and the jawline becomes less defined
- If large pores weren't a concern, you may now begin to notice them

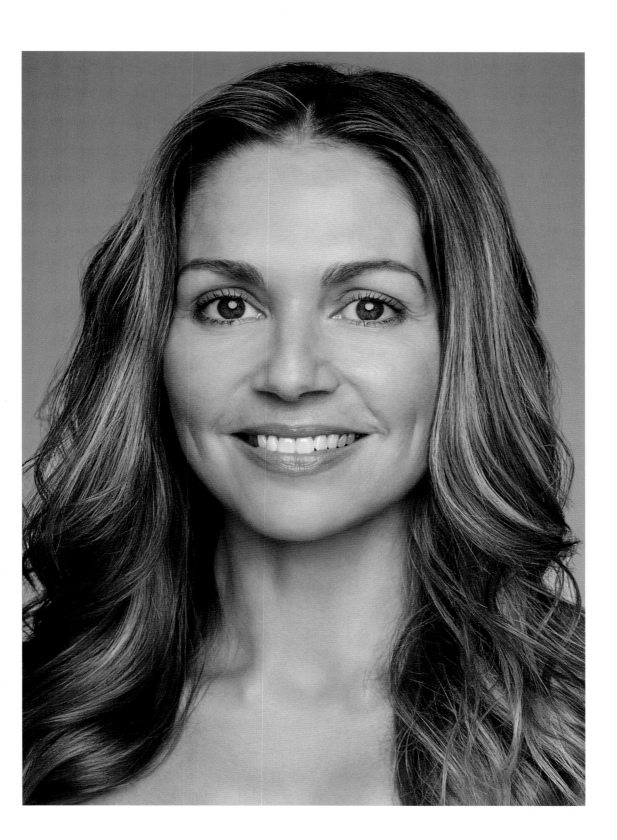

THE REALITY

Life is likely to be busy. You might be juggling the demands of work, children, family, ageing parents and bills. Yet now is also a time when you'll be more willing to take care of your complexion. If you step up your treatment focus you will see a real difference.

CHOOSING THE RIGHT PRODUCTS

Focus on home facial massage, weekly face masks, at-home peels and using skincare gadgets. Performing facial yoga and stretches on a daily basis will strengthen your face and neck muscles, keeping them supple and toned. This will lead to a more vibrant complexion. Use an exfoliating product or peel two or three times a week to smooth the texture of the skin and prevent dead skin cell build-up. Applying a higher strength retinol/vitamin A serum overnight will stimulate cell renewal and reduce the appearance of lines and wrinkles. A hyaluronic acid-based serum used during the day will deliver added moisture at a time when it's becoming increasingly dry. Vitamin C and antioxidant serums are also essential.

TIME FOR A PROFESSIONAL TREATMENT?

The main purpose of treatments at this age is to boost collagen production, increase cell turnover and support muscle tone. Look for microcurrent, LED, radiofrequency, Dermaroller, peels and oxygen therapies.

Do...

START LOOKING AFTER your neck and décolletage – your fifty-year-old self will thank you for it.

Think about ADDING in a vitamin A serum at night

MAKE EXFOLIATION part of your core routine.

Don't...

FORGET a daily SPF.

diet

A few small tweaks can make a big difference when it comes to re-energising and repairing your skin.

HORMONE-BALANCING FOODS

- Kidney support/liver cleansing: aim to drink 1.5 to 2 litres of water a day, between meals so that it doesn't dilute your digestive juices. If you find it boring to drink plain water, I recommend adding: peppermint, a slice of lemon, lime, orange, cucumber, celery or watermelon.

- Colon cleanse: increase your intake of fermented foods such as sauerkraut and kimchi.

- Foods high in fibre: flaxseed, nuts, oats, fruits, beans (such as black and kidney beans), pulses, apples, psyllium husks plus green leafy vegetables, brown rice, bran, chia seeds and garlic.

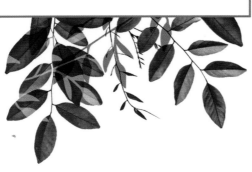

FIFTIES & BEYOND

Focus: strengthen, energise, repair & protect

Your 40s are good. Your 50s are great. Your 60s are fab. And 70 is fucking awesome.

HELEN MIRREN

At this age, the menopause may be giving you some skin concerns. Collagen production falls by around 30 per cent after the menopause, changing the skin's texture. It becomes thinner and more transparent, especially if you are very fair. Your neck and décolletage may show signs of ageing. Blood vessels are more sluggish, reducing the body's ability to deliver oxygen and nutrients to the dermis. This explains why our skin can lack radiance. The natural cushion of fat beneath the skin begins to lose its volume. The skin appears thinner and more fragile. When our bone density also begins to fall, the facial framework starts to shrink, causing the skin to look slack. Not forgetting the natural pull of gravity – especially visible around the jaw, eyes and cheeks. Pigmented patches may become more noticeable on the hands and face. I know all this sounds negative, but a few grey hairs and fine lines can be utterly beautiful and you should regard this as a time for positivity, confidence and freedom – breakouts should have passed and you can enjoy the liberation from the monthly hormonal cycle.

SKIN CHANGES
- Decline of collagen and elastin
- Fall in hyaluronic acid production
- Cholesterol build-up in the arteries of the dermis
- Volume of fat (subcutaneous tissue) thins, reducing the skin's underlying 'padding'
- Bone density shrinks the underlying facial framework
- Natural effect of gravity
- Melanin activity becomes impaired and pigmentation arises
- Facial muscles getting weaker

COMMON PROBLEMS
- Thinner skin
- Slower healing
- Hot flushes
- Rosacea and sensitivity
- Slackened muscle tone around the eyes, mouth, jaw and upper cheeks
- Dryness
- Deeper expression lines
- Loss of brightness
- Loss of plumpness
- Visible drop of contour around jaw, eyes, cheekbones and neck

- Sun spots
- Broken capillaries, especially on the cheeks

THE REALITY

Your children have flown the nest and hopefully you have more time on your hands and a greater expendable income. You're likely to be more confident. This is your time.

CHOOSING THE RIGHT PRODUCTS

Regular cleansing and moisturising are no longer sufficient, so focus on overnight treatments that deliver extra hydration in the form of serums and masks. Occasional home peels will help to smooth the skin, while richer moisturisers will keep it hydrated during the day. Look for products that have vitamins C and E combined, as they work in synergy with each other. Use an eye-specific retinol product at night and perform daily facial massage to tone and tighten the skin. Natural alternatives include using a floral water spritz to calm hot flushes. Rosewater is a good emotional supporter and excellent for calming sensitivity. Geranium balances hormones and is a great all-rounder for women.

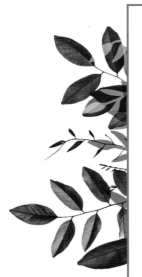

Do...

MOISTURISE, and lots of it

LOOK FOR thicker nourishing creams

IDEALLY have a facial every four to six weeks

MAKE THE MOST of home face massage

APPLY serums morning and evening

Don't...

FORGET eye creams

BE AFRAID of technology within face treatments, they can really help

FORGET weekly face masks for hydration

TIME FOR A PROFESSIONAL TREATMENT?

Opt for facial massage, microcurrent, manual lymphatic drainage (MLD), help with rosacea, LED, radiofrequency, Dermaroller, peels, oxygen and IPL for rosacea and broken capillaries.

KEEP ACTIVE

This is important, both physically and mentally, to maintain the vibrancy of your complexion. Go for low-impact activities such as hatha yoga, tai chi, walking, cycling and swimming.

diet

What we eat can affect the condition of our skin at every age and a few small tweaks can make a big difference

EAT MORE OF

- Essential fats to keep your skin nourished from the inside and counterbalance the drop in oestrogen impacting on hydration. This means flax, sesame, sunflower and pumpkin seeds.

- Phytoestrogens found in alfalfa, linseeds, beans, oats, fennel, celery, parsley and rhubarb.

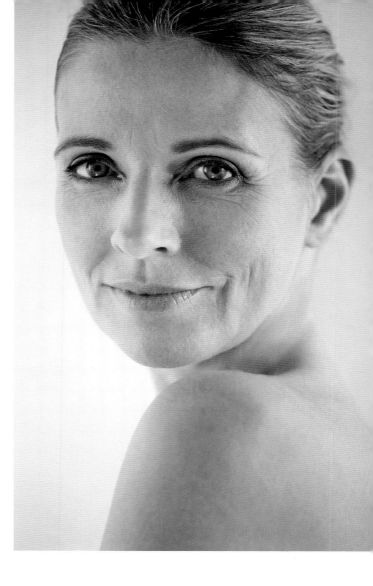

Skin is not intended to be perfectly porcelain and flawless. Freckles, age spots and lines show our life and character; they show that our skins are different and real without Instagram filters or airbrushing!

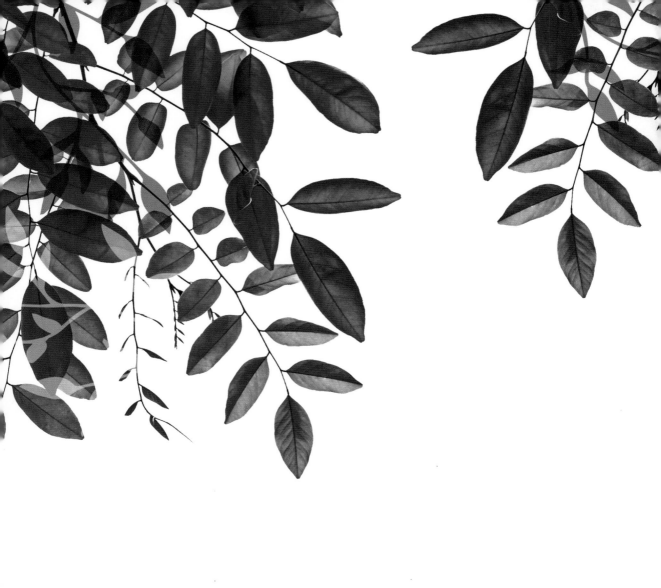

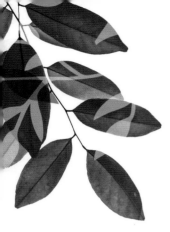

FOUR

SKIN TYPES & CONDITIONS

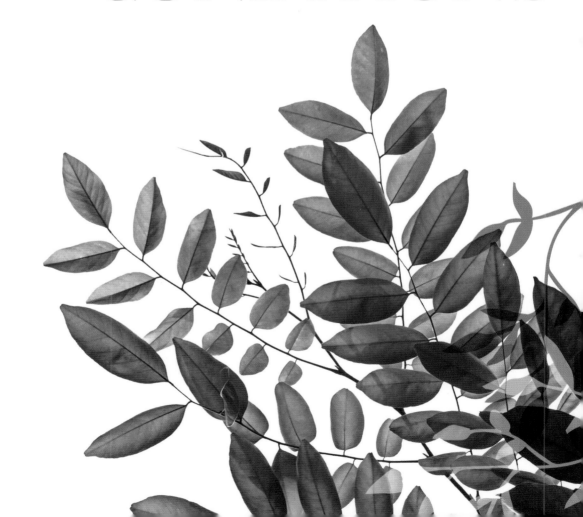

SKIN TYPES

The very first product I purchased was undoubtedly wrong for me. I chose it for its colour and pretty packaging, rather than whether it was best for my skin type. The wrong products can cause more problems than they fix, so selecting those that are right for your skin is essential.

Understanding your skin type is the way to do this. Our genes determine our skin type but lifestyle factors such as diet, stress levels and where you live affect the skin. I give clients a skin consultation to help identify their skin type and its condition.

This chapter is about equipping you with the skills to assess your skin at home. Bear in mind that most people have a combination of skin types.

I'm not beautiful like you.
I'm beautiful like me.

MARILYN MONROE

Normal skin

As a general rule, this complexion type is one that's resilient to external lifestyle factors and isn't giving you much cause for concern.

THE CHARACTERISTICS
- An even tone
- A soft, smooth texture
- Small pores with few or no blemishes
- No greasy patches or dry areas
- Only occasional hormonal spots

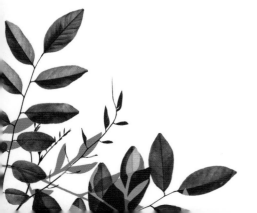

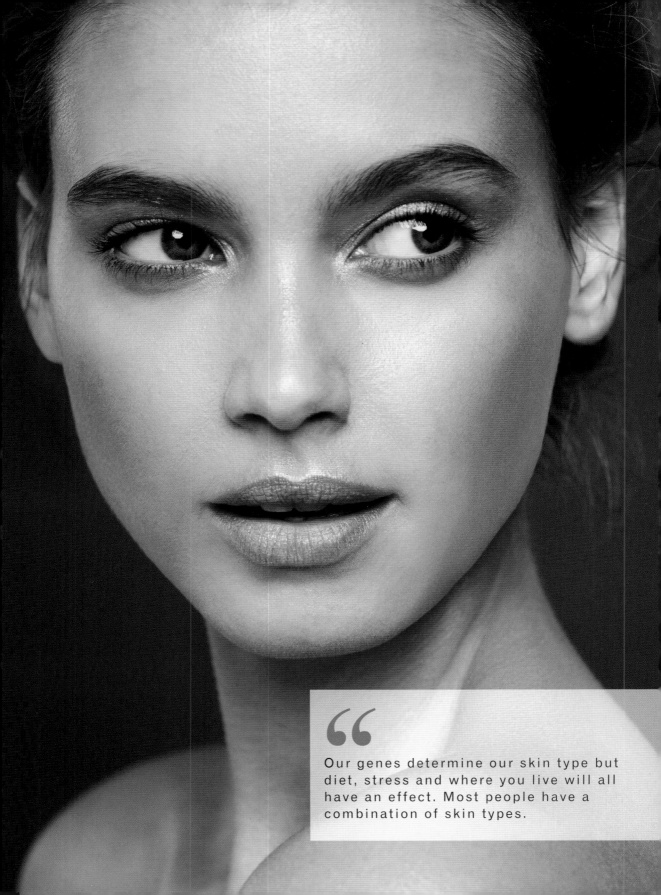

> " Our genes determine our skin type but diet, stress and where you live will all have an effect. Most people have a combination of skin types.

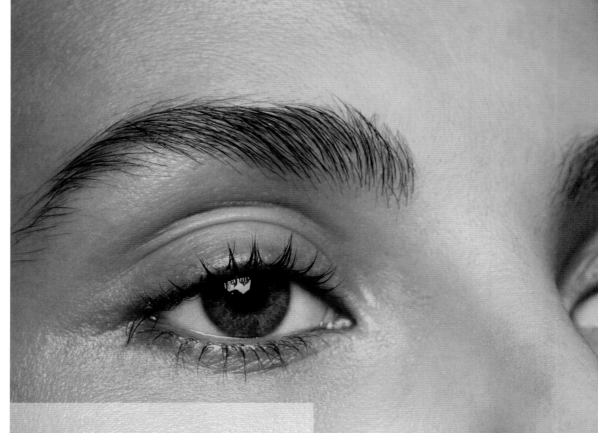

Combination skin

You're likely to have dry patches on the cheeks, mouth and around the eyes – and slightly oilier areas on the forehead, nose and chin (the 'T-zone').

When it comes to choosing products, combination skin can be a little frustrating. Should you select deep-cleansing products to combat the oiliness but make your dry patches drier? Or pick hydrating products for the dry patches that might bring you out in T-zone spots?

THE CHARACTERISTICS
- Slightly larger pores in the T-zone area
- Occasional dryness
- Occasional spots

Dry skin

More often than not, we inherit dry skin. It has a fine, dry texture with almost no visible pores. Although people with dry skin often have a lovely, porcelain complexion, it can feel rather uncomfortable and tight. The lack of natural oils being secreted on to the skin surface means fine lines and wrinkles may appear earlier. Simply drinking more water won't 'cure' dry skin. Balancing its oil content is a much more effective way of combating dryness.

THE CHARACTERISTICS
- Fine or invisible pores
- Sensitivity and redness
- A feeling of tightness
- Fine lines appear earlier
- Minimal oiliness
- A dull tone
- A flaky or rough texture

WHAT IRRITATES IT?
- Overly harsh skincare products
- Sun exposure
- Soap
- Chemicals such as chlorine
- Medication
- Depletion of hormones as we age

HOW TO MAKE THE MOST OF IT
Best products: balm, cream and oil cleansers and hydrating serums that contain ingredients such as hyaluronic acid and vitamin E. Exfoliate weekly to keep the dry skin surface smooth and add in face oils daily.

Best foods: a drier skin will benefit from internally hydrating foods, such as oils, nuts, seeds, flaxseed, linseeds, avocados, essential fatty acid and omega oil supplements and fish oils.

Dehydrated skin

This is often confused with dry skin. If your skin is dehydrated, it means that it's lacking in water. The skin is the very last organ to benefit from the water we drink and when we have this condition, moisture evaporates too quickly up through its layers. Its natural barrier function is weakened, making it even more prone to environmental damage.

THE CHARACTERISTICS
- Tightness
- Fine lines and a crepey texture
- A lack of radiance
- Loss of elasticity

WHAT IRRITATES IT?
- Harsh cleansing
- Insufficient protective skincare products
- Illness
- Not drinking enough water
- Air conditioning
- Extremes of hot and cold

HOW TO MAKE THE MOST OF IT
Best products: opt for a cream, milk or balm cleanser and include a serum containing hyaluronic acid and aloe vera, which is super-hydrating. Layer a gentle facial toner under your moisturiser. Weekly hydrating masks.

Best foods: watermelon, coconut water, celery and cucumber are all rich in hydration. Support the building blocks of the skin with oils, found in flaxseed and walnuts. Ensure you're drinking enough water.

Oily skin

If your skin is oily, you probably have coarse pores and are prone to developing blackheads and spots. The sebaceous (oil-producing) glands are overactive. The good news is that you're less likely to suffer from premature ageing!

THE CHARACTERISTICS
- Larger, more visible pores
- Shiny skin
- Thicker skin
- Blackheads and spots

WHAT IRRITATES IT?
Over-stripping skin with harsh chemical cleansers can cause excessive dryness, which sends a message to the sebaceous glands to produce more oil. You find yourself unable to break the spot-causing cycle. Please don't be seduced by the latest 'miracle' anti-ageing cream. It's likely to be far too rich and thick and will probably foster more breakouts.

HOW TO MAKE THE MOST OF IT
Best products: applying a 'dry' plant oil such as safflower (see chapter five) in very small amounts (about the size of half a pea) can help rebalance an over-oily skin by telling it that there's already oil present. I recommend using an oil, rather than a moisturiser, at night time for this reason.

The size of your pores is entirely dependent on genetics. There's not a single product that will reduce their size. I recommend that you choose a light-textured or oil-free moisturiser and make the most of light serums rather than relying on heavy moisturisers for hydration, as these will further block pores.

Sensitive skin

Everyone can suffer from sensitive skin from time to time. I find there are two types:

1. **REACTIVE:** a rash, inflammation, dryness or area of irritation that is often a histamine reaction (the body's natural response to a substance it doesn't like or has an allergy to).

2. **RESPONSIVE:** prone to flushing and sensitive to massage or changes in temperature. This is more of a blood-flow response, which causes pinkness and possible broken capillaries.

THE CHARACTERISTICS
- Patches of blotchy redness
- Thin, translucent skin
- Can be congested and blemished
- Some broken capillaries
- Rashes that come and go

WHAT IRRITATES IT?
- Temperature extremes
- Skincare ingredients
- Chemicals
- Synthetic fragrance
- Food allergies

Products to avoid: anything synthetically fragranced. Be careful, also, of exfoliants as these could cause the skin to flaire. Some aromatherapy oils will be too stimulating and worsen an irritated skin.

Food and drink to avoid: coffee and alcohol. If you have psoriasis, avoid the nightshade family of vegetables, which means peppers, potatoes, tomatoes and aubergine.

Best foods: anti-inflammatory foods such as turmeric, liquorice and cinnamon (see chapter eight), omega oils – flaxseed and hemp oil, and foods rich in B vitamins – brewer's yeast, oatmeal and legumes.

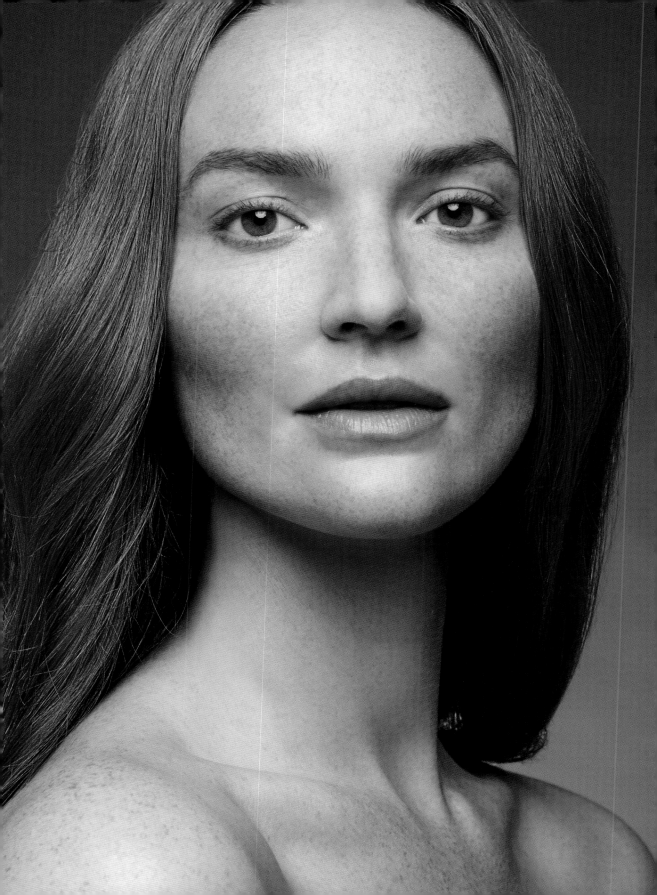

Your SKIN TONE

Your skin tone (colour) is different to your skin type. The pigment melanin determines its tone. Melanin helps protect it from sun damage. Professionals assess skin tone by using the Fitzpatrick scale, developed by Thomas Fitzpatrick in 1975, which helps us rate skin colour and see how different tones respond to the sun's rays. It also takes into consideration your eye and hair colour and how easily you tan. The scale goes from type 1, which always burns and never tans, to type 6, which very rarely burns and tans easily.

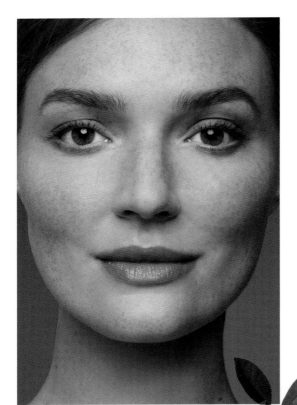

There are many variations, but here are just a few to give you an idea.

- **FAIR (CAUCASIAN): Fitzpatrick type 1 and 2**
Contains little melanin and is more susceptible to skin damage, premature ageing from sun exposure, broken veins, capillaries and rosacea, will always burn. Eye colour may be blue or grey. SPF 30–50 daily.

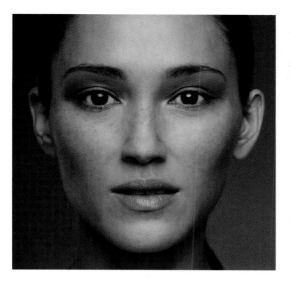

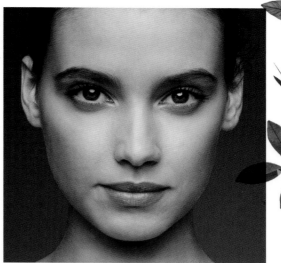

- **LIGHT BROWN & YELLOW:** Fitzpatrick type 3
Contain more melanin than white skin, so are more resistant to sun damage, can easily burn but may tan with care. Eye colour likely to be hazel or light brown. **SPF 30–50 daily.**

- **OLIVE:** Fitzpatrick type 4
Contains more melanin than white skin, so is less vulnerable to sun damage and tans easily. It also tends to be more elastic, so is less prone to premature ageing and stretch marks. **SPF 15–30 daily.**

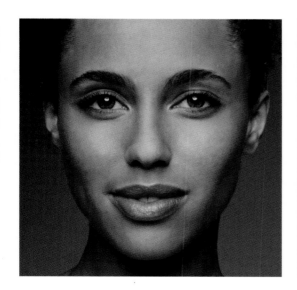

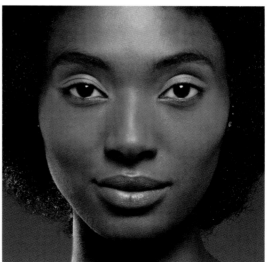

- **BROWN:** Fitzpatrick 4 and 5
Contains a greater density of sebaceous glands so tends to be oilier and ages more slowly. It is generally more elastic and stays firmer for longer. Eye colour likely to be brown. **SPF15+ daily.**

- **BLACK:** Fitzpatrick 5 and 6
It's the most resistant to sun damage, but is still susceptible to skin cancer, and needs longer in the sun to create the same levels of vitamin D as fair skin. Prone to dryness and keloid scaring (visible scars on the surface of the skin). Eye colour dark brown. **SPF 15 when in the sun.**

SKIN CONDITIONS

Acne

There are many factors that can spark and irritate acne, but the underlying issue is almost always hormones.

Originally a condition that plagued our teenage years, there's something of an adult acne epidemic spreading right now with people in their twenties, thirties and forties suffering from it. It might surprise you to know that up to 80 per cent of the population suffers from acne at some point. But why?

The sebaceous (spot-causing) glands are incredibly sensitive to hormonal fluctuations and easily become inflamed. The result is acne on the face, upper arms, back and chest. For most people, it begins in puberty when the body starts to produce hormones called androgens that stimulate the sebaceous glands. The link between acne and hormones means that women often suffer from recurrences during pregnancy, the menopause or when taking hormonal contraceptives.

Unfortunately, there's also an abundance of hidden hormone-disrupting chemicals present in our modern lives, including phthalates and plasticisers. These cause irreversible hormonal changes in men and women. Artificial fragrances are another form of irritant that disrupt the immune system – and make the skin less able to withstand attacks from spot-inducing bacteria.

THE LIFE CYCLE OF A SPOT

We have around five million hair follicles in our bodies, which is where spots start. Each tiny hole contains cells and glands that produce oil to help keep the skin plump and conditioned. But when there are too many cells or they become sticky as a result of hormones kicking in, they form a blockage. As more and more cells and sebum get trapped, the follicle starts to swell. The oxygen supply to the follicle also becomes reduced, producing the ideal environment for bacteria to thrive. Soon a spot is formed and the opening of the hole becomes blocked.

PROFESSIONAL TREATMENTS

Depending on the root cause of your acne, the efficacy of treatments can vary. Taking a combined approach with your home skincare regimen, professional treatments and diet will yield the best results. Blue LED light and laser treatments will kill the bacteria. Skin peels, focusing on reducing inflammation and targeting the bacteria, can be supportive, but a course is always needed to see results.

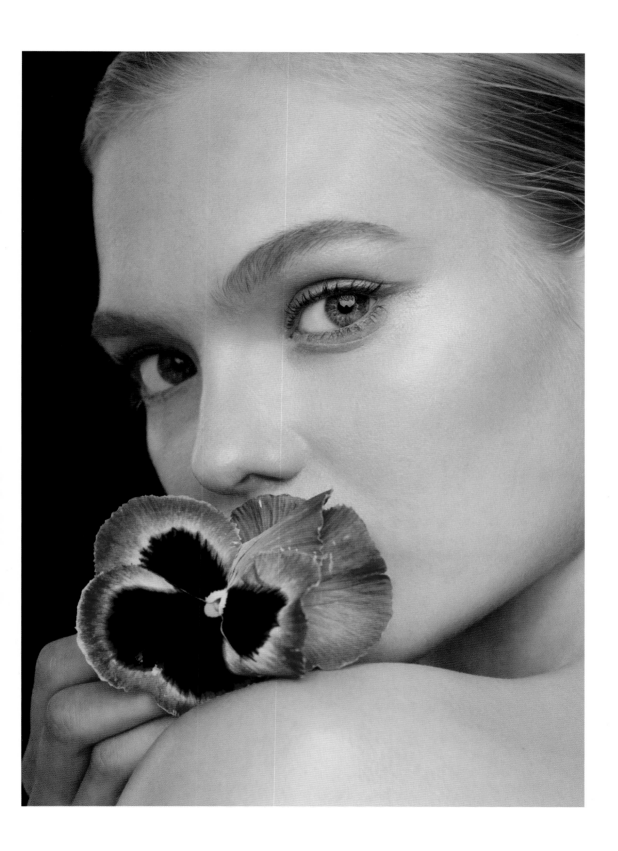

THE FOOD—ACNE LINK

By making subtle changes to your diet and taking certain supplements, you can do a huge amount to manage your acne.

• **Sugar:** there is medical evidence to suggest that ingesting just 100g of sugar can reduce your immune system's ability to function by as much as 50 per cent for up to five hours. Sugary foods reduce your body's ability to fight off infection, thereby increasing its risk of inflammation and acne. While a healthy immune system can heal a pimple in five to seven days, an immune system weakened by sugar won't be able to combat the inflammation underlying your spots, meaning it may ripen for ten days – or even two weeks.

• **Refined carbohydrates:** these cause a surge in the production of insulin inside the body. This can lead to an excess of male hormones, which stimulate the sebaceous glands. So try to limit your intake of sweet and starchy foods such as rice, pasta, bread, cereals, fruit and fruit juices, milk and milk products.

• **Meat:** meat contains hormones and hormone-like substances which can affect our body's balance internally. Alarmingly, dermatologists have reported that women who regularly eat red meat are more likely to suffer from acne and hirsutism.

• **Dairy:** see chapter eight.

foods *that* can help

ESSENTIAL FATTY ACIDS (EFAs): research has shown that EFAs can help regulate the hormonal imbalances that lead to acne. People with hormone-related acne have been shown to have deficiencies of EFAs. Good sources include flaxseed, hempseed, walnuts, dark green vegetables, pumpkin seeds, salmon, mackerel, sardines, anchovies, herring and tuna.

ZINC: oysters, shellfish, turkey, eggs, chickpeas, lentils, Brazil nuts, turnips, pumpkin seeds, oats, parsley, ginger root, buckwheat and carrots.

VITAMIN A: chili peppers, parsley, papaya, carrots,

mangoes, peaches, kale, apricots, pumpkin, sweet potatoes, broccoli and squash.

SOLUBLE FIBRE: flaxseed, nuts, oats, fruits, beans (such as black and kidney beans), pulses and apples.

INSOLUBLE FIBRE: green leafy vegetables, fruit skins, brown rice, bran, cabbage, chia seeds and garlic.

VITAMIN C: sweet potatoes, bell peppers, watercress and broccoli.

VITAMIN E: avocado, wheatgerm, pumpkin seeds and oily fish.

Top tips to clear acne...

1 CLEVER CLEANSING
If you suffer from acne, it's common to feel that the skin is 'dirty' and needs stringent cleaning. But acne isn't caused by dirt. Rather, the walls of a pore stick together deep within the skin. Choose a cleanser containing a combination of anti-inflammatory, antibacterial, antioxidant and hydrating ingredients. Salicylic acid, green tea, tea tree, retinoids, azelaic acid, alpha-hydroxy acid (AHA) and beta-hydroxy acid (BHA) will also exfoliate the skin and prevent sebum building up. Have another gentle cleanser to use on days when you feel your skin needs a 'rest'.

2 TRY NATURAL
Your skincare may be aggravating your condition, so try a product detox or natural approach. Aromatherapy lavender, rosemary, tea tree, frankincense and chamomile oils reduce inflammation and bring antibacterial benefits.

3 PUT AWAY THE MAGNIFIER
It only makes the problem look worse than it is – and please don't pick.

4 THE SUN
In the past, acne sufferers had been advised to take sunbeds to help. These days we're all much more aware of the dangers of overexposure to UV light, so this is not a form of treatment I would ever recommend.

5 MAKE-UP
Look for mineral make-up. I know you want to cover up but too many synthetics might clog pores further. Regularly wash your make-up brushes.

6 OILS
Use a tiny amount of oil at night time – your skin still needs oils to be healthy and balance itself.

7 SUPPORTING YOUR GUT
This is essential (see chapter eight).

Supplements to soothe

ZINC: helps repair scar tissue.

VITAMIN C: supports collagen production and skin repair.

VITAMIN E: increases skin tone, hydration and elasticity.

VITAMIN A: helps repair skin.

FLAXSEED: reduces inflammation and helps balance hormones.

" Stress reduces our skin's ability to heal wounds by around 40 per cent, so any spots you develop take longer to recover.

Milia

Milia look like tiny white bumps on the surface of your skin and are often found beneath the eyes and on top of cheekbones.

They form when dead skin cells and keratin become trapped between the layers of the epidermis. A fine layer of skin grows over the top of them, preventing them from sloughing off naturally. Milia aren't harmful but they can be a nuisance. In very rare cases, an autoimmune or genetic condition may be the underlying cause.

PROFESSIONAL TREATMENT:
This should definitely be left to professionals. They'll use a small probe or sterile needle to remove milia safely.

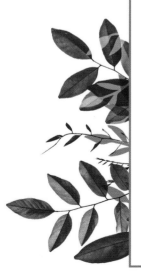

Do...

- **Cleanse:** twice daily with a good cleanser and a muslin cloth.

- **Exfoliate:** a peel containing lactic acid, AHAs or BHAs will slough off dead cells and prevent them becoming trapped beneath a 'lid' of growing skin.

- **Massage:** massaging the area around your milia will improve circulation and encourage trapped cells to become looser.

- **Retinol:** consider adding a gentle retinol product to your night-time routine to speed up skin cell turnover.

Don't...

- **Pick:** however tempting it is, picking will only ever end in tears. You're likely to damage the skin and possibly cause scarring. So resist!

- **Use heavy moisturisers:** an anti-ageing cream that's too rich for your skin makes it more likely to become blocked. Try a lighter oil or serum instead.

- **Use products containing mineral oil and silicones:** these create a barrier on the surface of the skin, which exacerbates milia.

Rosacea

This skin disorder results in facial flushing, redness and sensitivity across the cheeks, nose, chin and forehead.

Rosacea can also affect the scalp, eyes, ears, neck and back. The flushing and redness relate to the vascular blood supply and the inflammation of the sebaceous (oil) glands, which causes pimples, red bumps and uneven skin texture. It can occur at any age, but I find it to be most common amongst women of thirty to fifty years old. Unfortunately, the root cause still isn't known, though recent research suggests that a microscopic mite called Demodex that exists on all of us may be a contributing factor.

MEDICAL TREATMENT:
Prescribed oral antibiotics can offer some relief but usually symptoms return. Gut health is closely connected to the health of the skin, so probiotics are essential to counterbalance the impact on the gut of antibiotics. Topical medication, usually in the form of antibacterial, anti-fungal creams, often works for a short period of time, although some people find that they merely exacerbate the problem.

ROSACEA TRIGGERS
We have chemicals called histamines inside our body's cells. When these are released into the bloodstream, in what's known as a 'histamine response', they cause itching and flushing.

• **Food:** As certain foods contain histamines and trigger this release, it's best to avoid them if you suffer from rosacea. Bananas, cheese,

tomatoes, chocolate, canned tuna, avocado, jam, yogurt, strawberries and pineapple can all bring on flushing. Alcohol, hot drinks, caffeine, spicy foods, citrus fruit, smoked foods, vinegar and soy sauce are also common triggers of rosacea.

• **Stress:** Stress sets rosacea off, which in turn affects our self-esteem, making us feel even more stressed-out.

• **Weather:** Both extremes of temperature and the sun's rays can bring on skin flushing. Some chemicals in sunscreen can also act as a trigger, so take care to choose an SPF based upon zinc oxide or titanium dioxide, which are kinder to sensitive skin.

• **Skincare products:** My clients who suffer from rosacea usually have hypersensitive skin that reacts to many conventional creams containing fragrance and colours.

• **Medication:** Some prescription can cause flare-ups. If you have a history of long term use of antibiotics this can be a contributing factor.

NATURAL TREATMENTS:
Lymphatic massage can be effective. Flushing causes fluid and toxins to accumulate within the skin. By having regular lymphatic face treatments, you can help keep this build-up of toxins to a minimum.

the right products

You will benefit from choosing organic products as they contain fewer or no synthetic ingredients which aggravate the condition. Look for calming ingredients such as chamomile, calendula, aloe vera and chickweed. Oils that are particularly good include blackcurrant seed oil, sweet almond oil, evening primrose oil, rosehip seed oil, sea buckthorn and hemp seed.

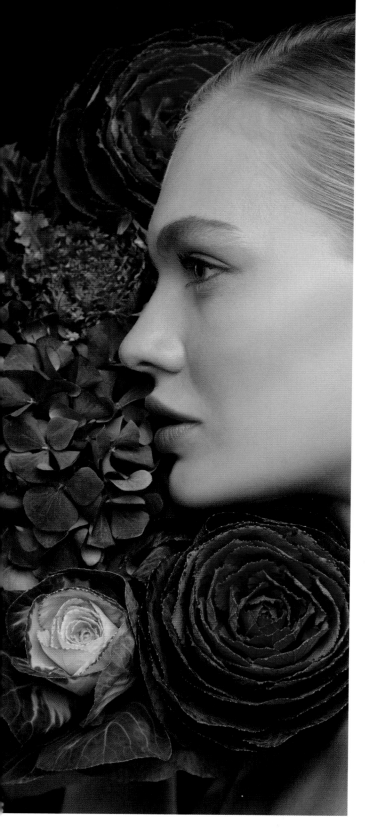

4 tips to beat rosacea

1 ### HERBAL TEAS
Sage, rosemary, thyme, chamomile, lemon balm, milk thistle, fennel, garlic and marshmallow root.

2 ### EXERCISE
Strenuous exercise can bring on flushes. I suggest low-impact, such as walking, Pilates, yoga, cycling. Avoid chlorinated swimming pools as this will only irritate it.

3 ### SUPPLEMENTS
Probiotics such as acidophilus can help keep the bacteria in the gut healthy.

4 ### MAKE-UP
Covering it with make-up can exacerbate the problem. Natural mineral make-up is less likely to irritate the skin.

And you can...

- Keep a facial spritz in your handbag or car. When you feel a flush coming on, you can use it to cool and soothe the skin.

- Suck on an ice cube – it cools the skin from the inside!

- It's best to avoid alcohol altogether, but if you want to have a drink, try gin or vodka with soda water and lemon rather than wine, which has sulphates and a higher sugar content.

Pigmentation

Hyperpigmentation develops when your skin produces too much melanin.

Sun exposure, hormones, pregnancy, the pill and certain medication can trigger this process. Unfortunately, once you've developed hyperpigmentation, it will return even after successful treatment because the DNA of our skin cells has been affected for ever. Fragrance, essential oils, antiseptics, acne medication and some prescription drugs can also make the skin more sensitive to the sun, so save your perfume for night time and ask your doctor about any medication you're taking.

DIFFERENT TYPES

• **Sun-induced age spots:** these are an inevitable part of ageing often found on the outer areas of the face and backs of your hands.

• **Hormonal pigmentation:** this is often referred to as 'melasma'. It usually occurs on the central areas of your face, the cheekbones, around the eyes, the central forehead and upper lip. Chloasma is the pigmentation that occurs in pregnancy, commonly known as the 'pregnancy mask'. It appears like a butterfly pattern across the face but usually fades when you finish breastfeeding.

• **Post-inflammatory pigmentation:** this occurs when there has been some type of trauma to the skin, such as acne scarring, burning and some laser treatments.

PROFESSIONAL TREATMENTS:
laser, Fraxel, IPL, kojic acid, skin peels, hydroquinone.

Skin cancer

Malignant melanoma is a serious type of skin cancer that occurs when the growth of pigment cells (our melanocytes) happens in a rapid, uncontrolled way.

SYMPTOMS
It can be difficult to tell the difference between a melanoma and a normal mole. The following checklist (known as the ABCDE list) will give you an idea of what to look out for.

THINK A,B,C,D,E
• A: Asymmetry.
Melanomas are likely to be irregular or asymmetrical, while ordinary moles are usually symmetrical.
• B: Border.
Melanomas are more likely to have an irregular border with jagged edges. Moles usually have a well-defined, regular border.
• C: Colour.
Melanomas tend to have more than one colour. They may have different shades of brown mixed with black, red, pink, white or a bluish tint. Moles are usually one shade of brown.
• D: Diameter.
Melanomas are usually more than 7mm in diameter. Moles are normally no bigger than the blunt end of a pencil (about 6mm across).
• E: Evolving (or changing).
Look for changes in the size, shape or colour of a mole.

If you notice any of the above signs or find that a mole is tingling or itching, it's best to get it checked.

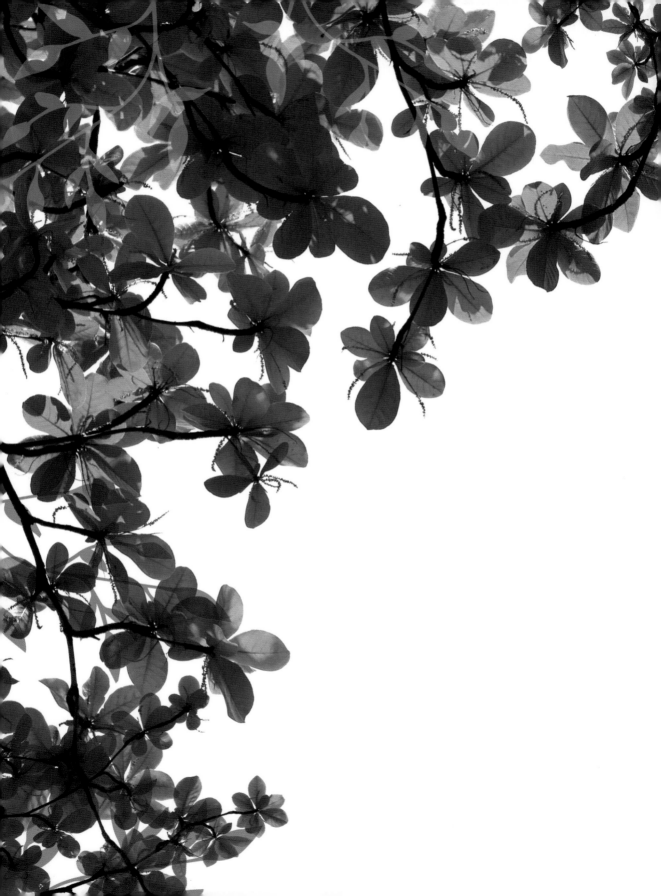

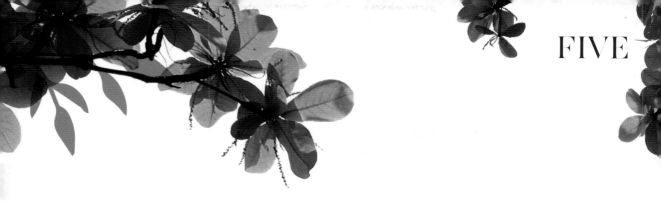

FIVE

BUILDING YOUR OWN BEST ROUTINE

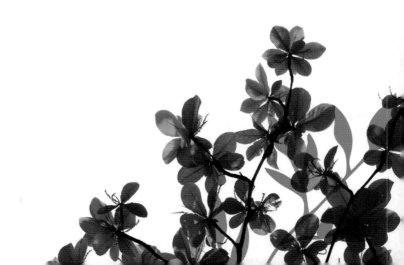

how to
MAKE YOUR PRODUCTS WORK *for you*

While our grandmothers' generation might have relied on soap, water and basic moisturiser, our expectations of looking younger are much higher now. Science and technology has moved on at an incredible pace, giving us all the potential to have great skin. The rows of 'miracle' creams, 'wonder' serums, lotions, masks and exfoliators in a beauty hall can be overwhelming. How are we supposed to choose the products that are right for us?

In order to make visible improvements and gain long-term benefits, you have to identify a combination of products that work together. The most expensive aren't necessarily the best. Their effectiveness will be determined by the quality of ingredients, how they're formulated, how well they're absorbed and how good a match they are with your skin.

the skincare system

You need to understand what order to apply the different products in to get the best results. As a general rule, I'd advise applying the product with the thinnest consistency first, then building towards the thickest textures. Remember to allow each product to sink in before applying the next.

- **THE MORNING ROUTINE**
  Before you begin your morning make-up routine, apply your products in the following order: **cleanser, toner, serum, eye cream, moisturiser, sun protection.**

- **THE BEDTIME RITUAL**
  Each night, apply your products in the following order:
  1. cleanser
  2. toner
  3. serum
  4. face oil or moisturiser

If you have oily skin, you could simply cleanse, tone and finish with serum or oil and definitely omit the moisturiser

- **THE PERFECT DOSE**
  This will vary slightly from one brand to another.

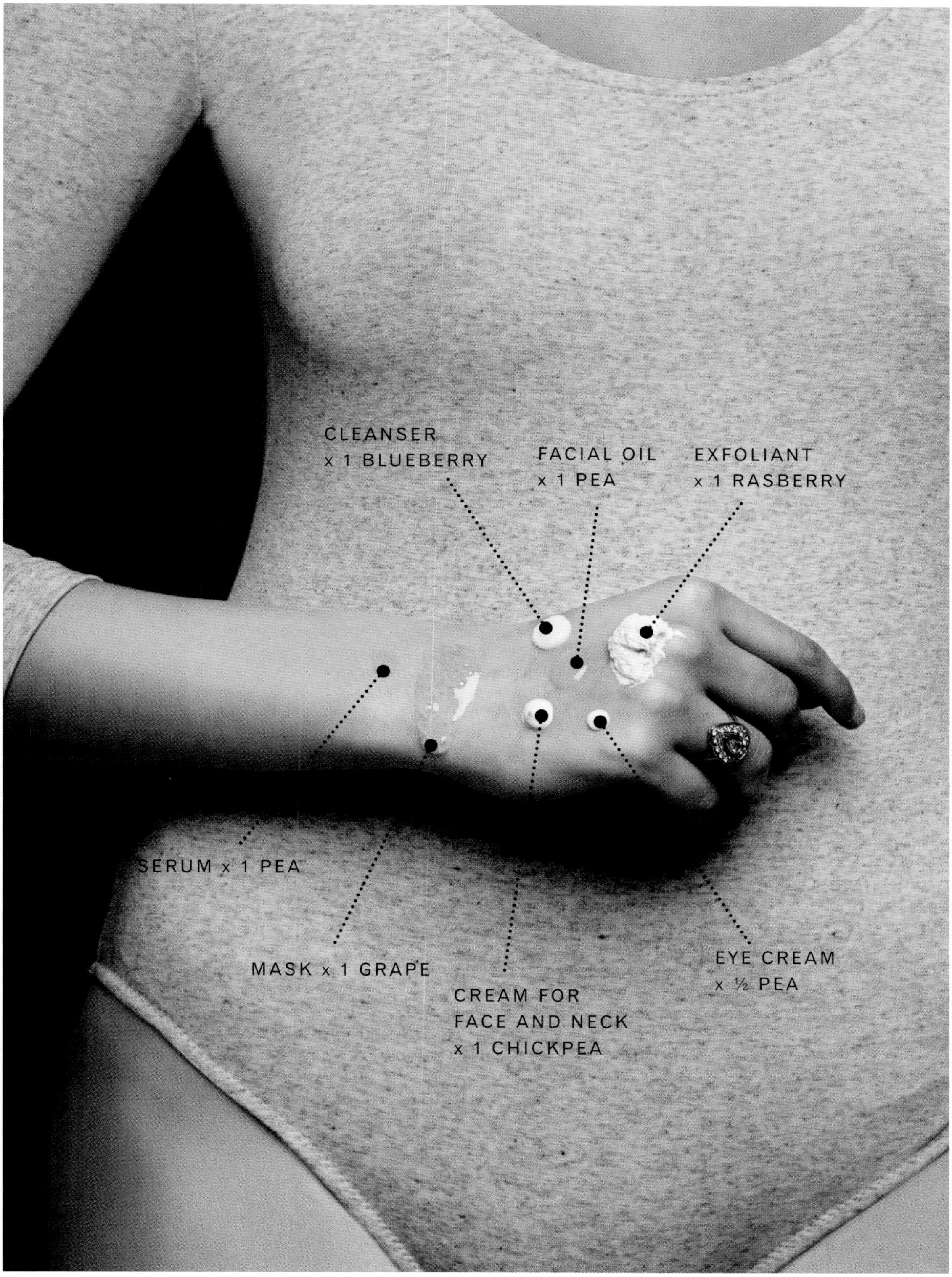

CLEANSER
x 1 BLUEBERRY

FACIAL OIL
x 1 PEA

EXFOLIANT
x 1 RASBERRY

SERUM x 1 PEA

MASK x 1 GRAPE

CREAM FOR
FACE AND NECK
x 1 CHICKPEA

EYE CREAM
x ½ PEA

Cleansers

Washing with water on its own can cause the skin to become dry but a good cleanser will remove surface dirt, bacteria, sweat and make-up to prevent the pores from becoming blocked. The massaging action we use when cleansing also helps bring fresh blood flow to the skin surface, making us look fresher and healthier. While too harsh a cleanser may cause dryness, choosing one that's too rich could trigger oiliness and breakouts. If your skin feels 'squeaky-clean' and tight after cleansing, it's a sign that your product might be too harsh for you.

Types of cleanser

The cleanser you choose will depend on your preference and skin condition. I like to have two to choose from, according to how my skin feels on any given day.

- **CREAM/MILK**

These offer a more soothing cleanse than a wash. Traditionally these were applied to cotton-wool pads and wiped over the face. I suggest putting some into the palm of your hand and working over your face, eyes and neck before removing it with water and a cotton or muslin cleansing cloth. These add an extra, gentle daily buffing to support the removal of dead skin cells for a brighter complexion.

- **FACE WASH**

Wash cleansers need to be mixed with water. Traditional foaming cleansers can be harsh, as the chemicals used to make them lather often have a drying effect. Avoid sodium lauryl sulfate (SLS) as it strips and dries and can make the skin sensitive. Some of the newer formulations contain gentler, plant-derived foaming agents that are a much better choice if you need a deeper cleanse.

- **BALMS**

These are often a gentle, nourishing blend of plant oils, essential oils and herbs that remove make-up – including mascara – easily as the oils 'melt' what's on the skin surface. After smoothing and massaging them over the skin, remove them with a warm muslin cloth to ensure no pore-blocking residues remain. Each balm will vary considerably due to the different blends of oils. I avoid mineral oils (petroleum, liquid paraffin) – they are safe but with long-term use pores become blocked, resulting in spots and skin becoming dull.

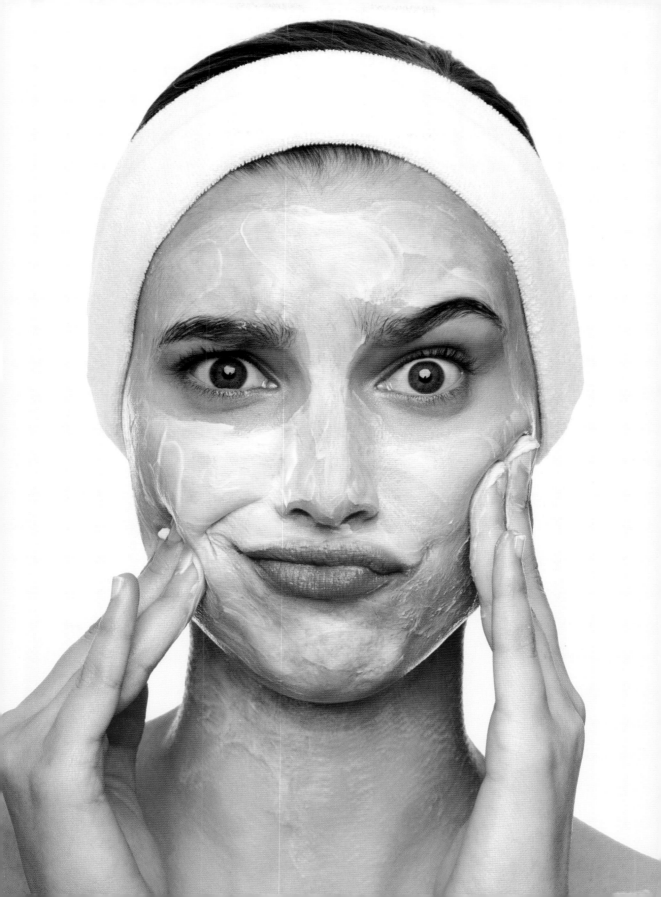

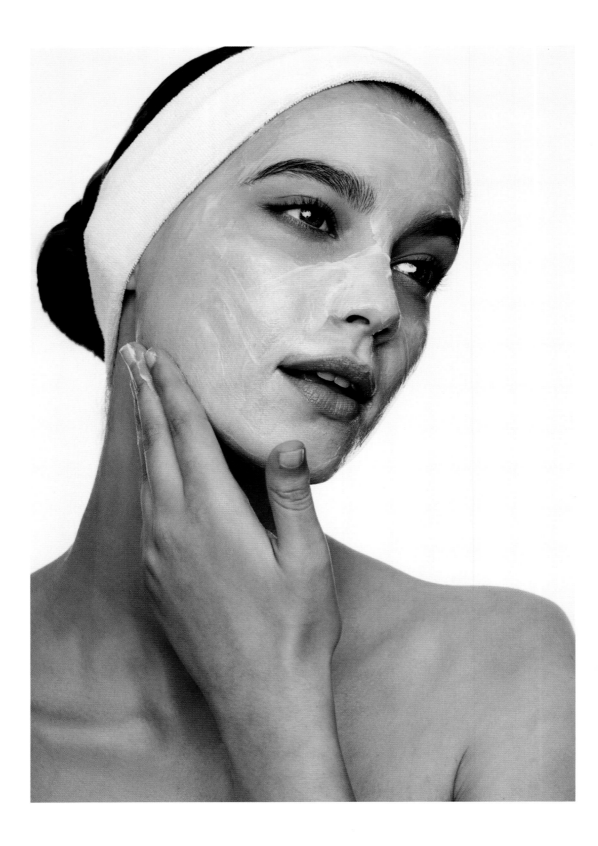

- **MELTING BALMS/OILS**

These represent a newer generation of cleanser. They generally come in a gel or oil consistency that transforms into a light milk when you add water. They're a great way to remove make-up and grime and are best removed using a muslin cloth.

- **FACE WIPES**

Even though they're convenient, I'd advise you to steer clear! They're usually packed with alcohol, synthetics and fragrance, which will irritate your skin, causing sensitivity and redness. Furthermore, they rarely provide an effective cleanse. Save them for festivals, travelling and when you're really super short on time.

- **MICELLAR WATERS**

These are a halfway house between a traditional cleanser and a toner that originate from France and are considered a simple, effective method of removing make-up and dirt in a gentle way without the need to wash off. They take their name from micelles, which are tiny round balls of cleansing oil molecules that float in water. Apply it to a cotton-wool pad and swipe it over the skin. You may need a second cleanse. I see these as a make-up remover rather than a proper cleanser; however they can be helpful for eczema and super-sensitive skins that need a really gentle cleanse.

Cleansing the clever way

- **TWICE A DAY**

Should we cleanse twice a day? The answer is yes! Whilst a night-time cleanse is essential to remove the make-up and grime of the day, it's also important to clean the skin when you wake up in the morning. Overnight the skin eliminates toxins via the pores, so starting the day with a clean canvas removes the toxic residue from the skin surface and will make the products you apply more easily absorbed and effective.

- **DOUBLE CLEANSING**

Use a cleanser to remove the uppermost make-up and surface grime, then another product or the same one again to perform a further, deeper cleanse. For the first cleanse I love using a cream or balm, followed by a gentle wash for the second.

5 steps to the perfect cleanse

1. Warm your cleanser between your palms.

2. Massage it into the face to stimulate blood flow and aid detoxification. Add water if necessary. Work around your whole face, using small circles over your chin and mouth and larger ones around your eyes. Don't forget your neck, behind the ears and décolletage.

3. Add warm water.

4. Remove the cleanser with a warm cloth.

5. Splash your face with cold water to close your pores and freshen up your complexion.

tip A collection of face cloths is essential to ensure so you have a fresh one to use every day.

Toners

Toners were traditionally a means of removing the residue left by cream cleansers. They contained high concentrations of alcohol and would often strip the skin, leaving it feeling dry and sensitive. Modern-day toners do have a place in your skincare routine, but you need to select one for your skin type based upon its key ingredients.

Types of toners

- **HYDRATING:** these contain aloe vera, vitamin E and cucumber.

- **SKIN BALANCING:** contain salicylic acid and/or witch hazel and hold antibacterial, anti-inflammatory benefits for the skin.

- **EXFOLIATING AND BRIGHTENING:** contain AHAs. Exfoliating toners are a water-based liquid that you use like a toner with cotton-wool pads; however they are not really toners but another way of exfoliating the skin.

HOW TO APPLY

After cleansing, apply your toner to the face using a cotton-wool pad. Some can be spritzed and left on the skin. Follow this with your serum and moisturiser. The right toner will help any products you apply afterwards penetrate more easily, bringing even better results.

Face serums are the powerhouse of your skincare routine.

Serums

Serums are the powerhouse of your skincare routine. Each will contain different active ingredients that have been chosen for their ability to target key concerns such as acne, ageing, hydration, redness and uneven pigmentation.

There's a serum for everyone and every skin concern! Serums have a lighter, more liquid texture than a moisturiser and a higher concentration of active ingredients that are absorbed faster and deeper into the skin. A moisturiser works predominantly on the surface of your skin to keep the upper layers plump, hydrated and protected. Serums are designed to be layered under a moisturiser, so that the two can work together and keep all layers of the skin healthy, balanced and youthful.

HOW TO APPLY

A little generally goes a long way. It's important to cleanse your skin before applying your serum – any oils remaining on the surface will slow down absorption and reduce the effectiveness of active ingredients. Serums can be used morning and night, depending on their key ingredients. If yours contains retinol save it for night time as your skin's sensitivity to sun exposure will be increased.

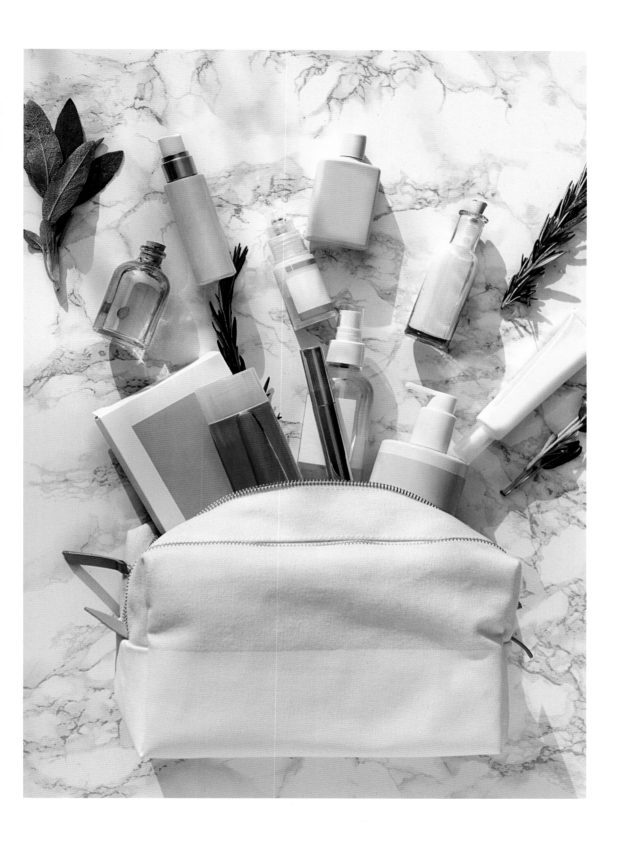

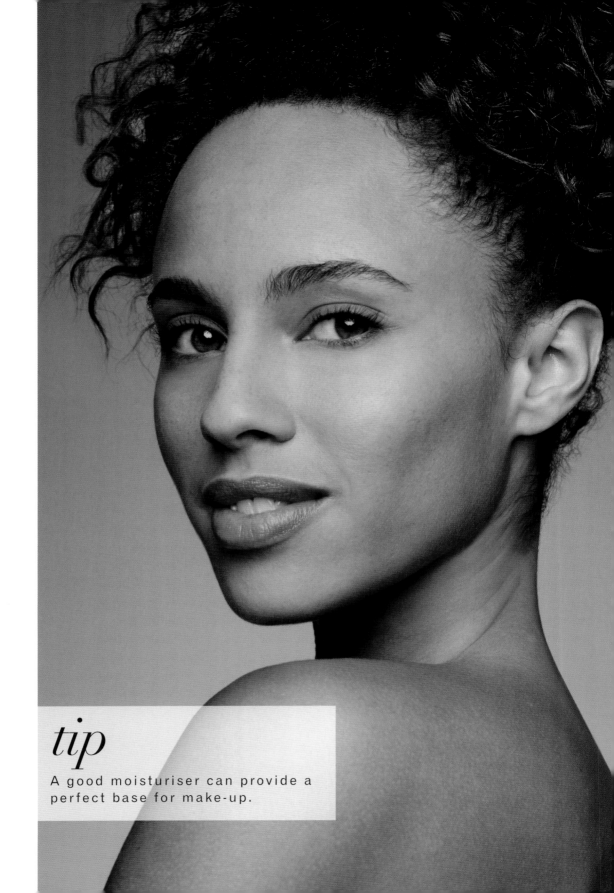

tip
A good moisturiser can provide a
perfect base for make-up.

Moisturisers

These are an essential part of our skincare routines. Their ability to multitask and address a number of skin issues means they're ideal for the demands of modern living. I like to think of a basic moisturiser like a mayonnaise mix of water and oil, with the skin requiring both to be healthy.

A good moisturiser can...

1 HELP maintain your skin's natural protective barrier and prevent water loss associated with external factors such as central heating, air conditioning and changes in weather patterns.

2 ACT as a cleaver humectant (it prevents moisture loss and takes moisture from the air to feed to your skin).

3 MAINTAIN the skin's natural moisturising factors (NMFs) – the mixture of amino acids and water-soluble salts inside your skin cells. Because these are water-soluble, they can easily be washed out, which reduces the cells' ability to hold on to their moisture, leaving your skin feeling dry.

4 PROVIDE a good base for make-up.

5 EVEN OUT dry patches and soften the appearance of fine lines.

6 FEED AND NOURISH the skin with key ingredients.

7 PROTECT the skin from environmental damage such as UV rays and pollution.

Moisturisers for different skin types

Your skin type and needs determine which moisturiser you should be using. If you have oily skin, you may choose an oil-free moisturiser in the morning to prevent your face from looking shiny during the day. On the other hand, if you have dry skin you might look for a richer texture.

- **DAY AND NIGHT MOISTURISERS**
  Traditionally, day creams are lighter than night creams, which tend to be thicker and richer. However, I see better results if this tradition is turned on its head. My preference is for richer day creams and much finer products for night application. Unless you have really dry or ageing skin, a rich night cream is likely to cause breakouts. Oily skins do not need a rich night cream.

- **BB AND CC CREAMS**
  These multitasking products originated in Germany and offer an affordable means of hydrating, sun protection and colour coverage all in one cream. In my view they fall into the 'make-up' category rather than 'skincare'. Use them as a means of linking your skincare routine with your make-up, rather than relying on them as a moisturiser or SPF.

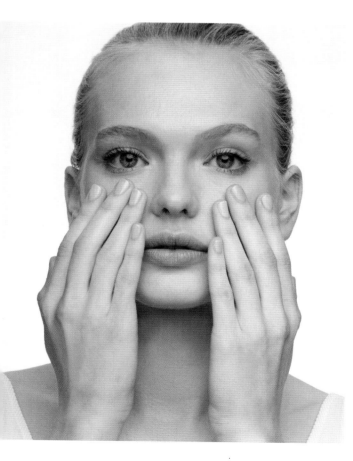

Exfoliators

These help remove dead and dull skin cells to create a smoother surface, and a brighter complexion, and help speed skin cell turnover.

There are two main types. Physical exfoliants have a gritty texture and contain particles that buff the skin surface and remove dead cells. The newer generation of exfoliators contain AHAs and BHAs that work by gently dissolving dead skin cells to smooth and refresh the skin. All skin types require different amounts of exfoliation. I would suggest a minimum of once a week, however thicker, oiler skin may require up to four times.

Be conscious of what hidden exfoliants you may have in your cleanser and serums as this will impact on your frequency of exfoliation.

Sun protection

I suggest wearing sun protection on your face all year round – even in winter. If you want to age your best, it's one of the skincare musts! Sun exposure is the biggest factor in premature ageing.

There are two main types of sun-protecting ingredients: physical and chemical.

CHEMICAL SUNSCREENS

These absorb and trigger a chemical reaction within the skin, which allows their protective mechanism to be activated. Apply them 20 minutes before going out in the sun while this process takes place. Chemical SPFs absorb the ultraviolet radiation energy within the skin and then 'break down' the sunlight to create their protective effect. Some commonly used chemical UV filters to look out for are octocrylene, avobenzone, octinoxate, octisalate, oxybenzone, homosalate and helioplex.

PHYSICAL SUNSCREENS

Physical sunscreens are usually made up of the minerals zinc oxide and titanium dioxide. They're generally considered safer than chemical sunscreens because they don't absorb into the skin and create a chemical reaction but sit on the surface and reflect the sun's rays. They are an effective way to block UVA and UVB rays, but because they're often thicker, they tend to leave a white film on the skin. Some brands that combine these minerals with oils have found a clever way to reduce this effect. Zinc oxide has mild healing properties and is safe for use on small children and very sensitive skin types. It's often used in nappy rash creams to support healing and also soothes blemishes.

WHAT AN SPF NUMBER MEANS

The higher the SPF number, the more protection your skin gets. If it takes 20 minutes of sun exposure for your skin to start turning red without sun protection, then applying an SPF 15 should theoretically allow you to be in the sun for 15 times longer before you burn. However, that would mean you can stay in the sun for an extra five hours. In reality, being in the midday sun with only an SPF 15 for five hours would most likely result in sunburn. Most sunscreens won't remain effective after two hours, so they need to be reapplied to maintain an adequate level of protection.

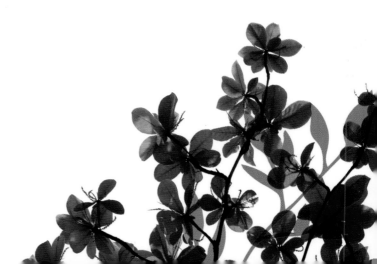

Masks

Few of us take the time to apply masks. Compared to dashing on a serum or moisturiser, waiting for something to work for 10 to 20 minutes seems like a lifetime! But masks are a game changer that many are missing out on. They are an integral part of a professional facial, so it makes sense that we should take these hard-working gems into our skincare routine at home.

Types of masks

Masks are targeted towards specific skin concerns and are often packed with more potent active ingredients than our regular moisturisers – so only need to be used once or twice a week to bring about fabulous results. The key is selecting the best mask for your skin.

You can do this by learning to match certain ingredients with your individual skin concern.

Here are a few to look out for:

- **PORE-CLEANSING MASKS:** clay, salicylic acid

- **HYDRATING MASKS:** aloe vera, plant oils, glycerin, shea butter, hyaluronic acid

- **EXFOLIATING MASKS:** AHAs, jojoba beads, nuts and seeds, fruit acids

- **BRIGHTENING MASKS:** AHAs, vitamin C

- **BALANCING MASKS:** aloe vera, cucumber, honey

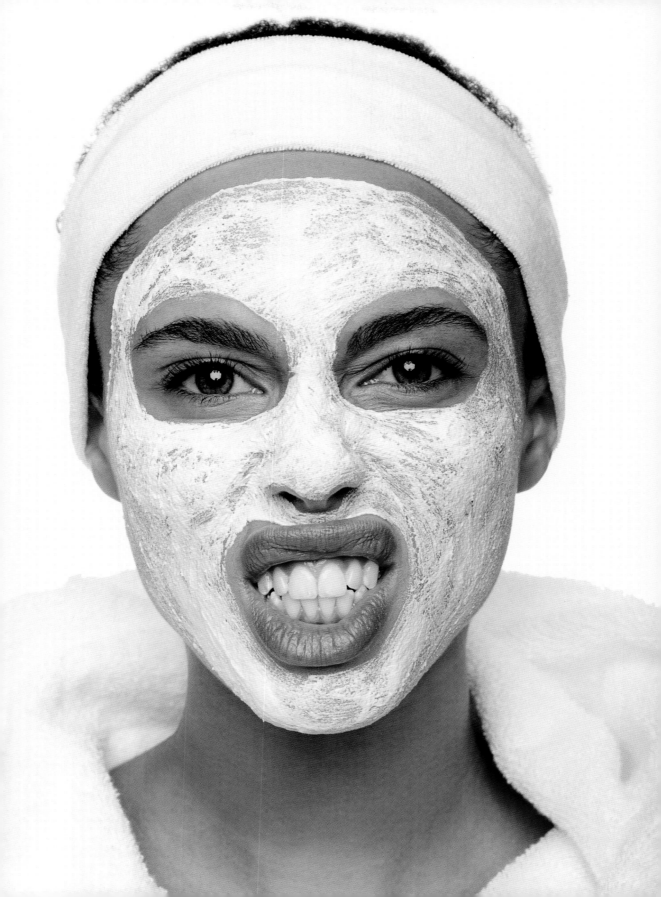

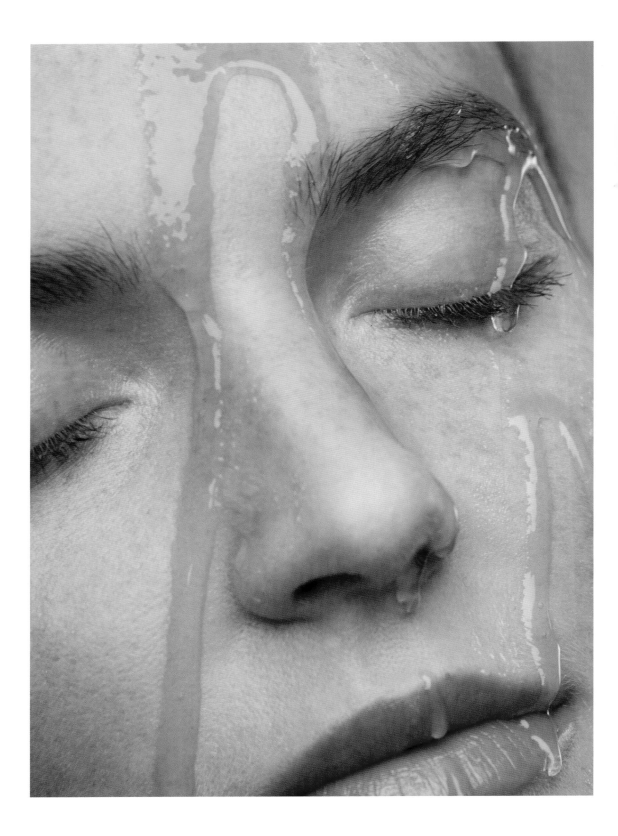

Oils

Plant oils bring multiple benefits. They replace oil that the skin has already lost and help prevent further moisture loss. Not only do they nourish but each oil will have differing skin benefits such as antioxidant, antibacterial and anti-inflammatory. Each oil has a different molecule size, meaning some penetrate deeper and quicker into your skin's layers than others.

Which one is best for you?

There are many beautiful blends of plant oils available, here are just a few that are good for particular skin types:

- **SENSITIVE SKIN:** sweet almond, peach kernel, evening primrose, St. John's wort, avocado

- **AGEING SKIN:** argan, rosehip seed, camellia, sea buckthorn, pomegranate seed

- **COMBINATION SKIN:** borage, pomegranate, rosehip seed, sea buckthorn

- **OILY SKIN:** look for 'dry oils', which have a lighter texture, absorb quickly and are similar to the skin's own sebums – such as moringa, apricot kernel, olive oil, safflower, hemp, borage, milk thistle.

Avoid anything containing mineral oils, synthetics or petroleum oil as they have very little if any nourishing skin benefit, unless you have broken skin, which requires a more waterproof, protective barrier.

HOW TO APPLY

The texture of oils makes them perfect for massaging in. This will not only help them sink deeper into the skin, but also give you a fresh, healthy glow by bringing fresh blood to the surface and helping drain puffiness. Oils can be used day and night – I love the evening to support the skin's natural regeneration process that occurs when we sleep. Only a small pea-sized amount is necessary – any more may leave the skin greasy. Oils don't require added preservatives because bugs generally won't grow in them, which makes them purer. However, if left in sunlight and aged they can go rancid and will increase free-radical damage when applied to the skin.

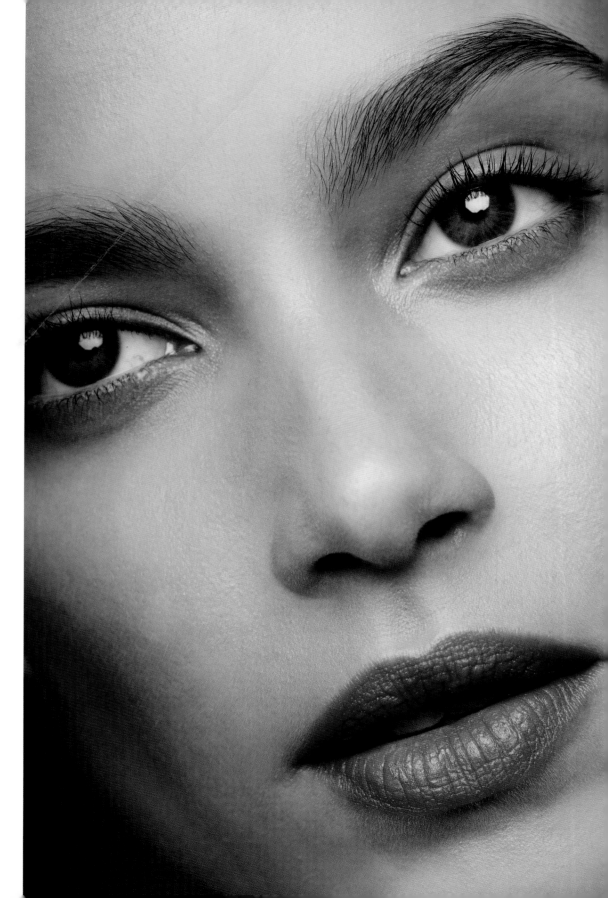

eye products

Eye creams are an essential part of your routine from the age of thirty plus and their formulas will be specifically designed to focus on this delicate area. The skin around the eyes is often the first to show signs of the ageing process as it's ten times finer than on the rest of our face. The muscles underlying this skin are also the most active in your body. So it's particularly vulnerable to developing lines, wrinkles and puffiness.

Getting the best from them

- Tap the eye cream or serum around the whole eye area. Most formulas will be safe to apply over the eyelids, an often forgotten area that gets increasingly crepey as we age.

- Apply eye creams in the morning rather than when you go to bed. While we sleep creams can sit in the delicate skin around our eyes because our eyelids are closed and our circulation has slowed, so they can make you look more tired and puffy when you wake.

- Applying your eye cream just before your concealer will make a huge difference to how your make-up sits and feels on the skin. Fine lines will be less noticeable and your concealer won't sink into the eye creases.

- Apply serums or gels in the evening.

- To double up and supercharge your eye care, try applying a retinol eye product at night and a hydrating cream in the day.

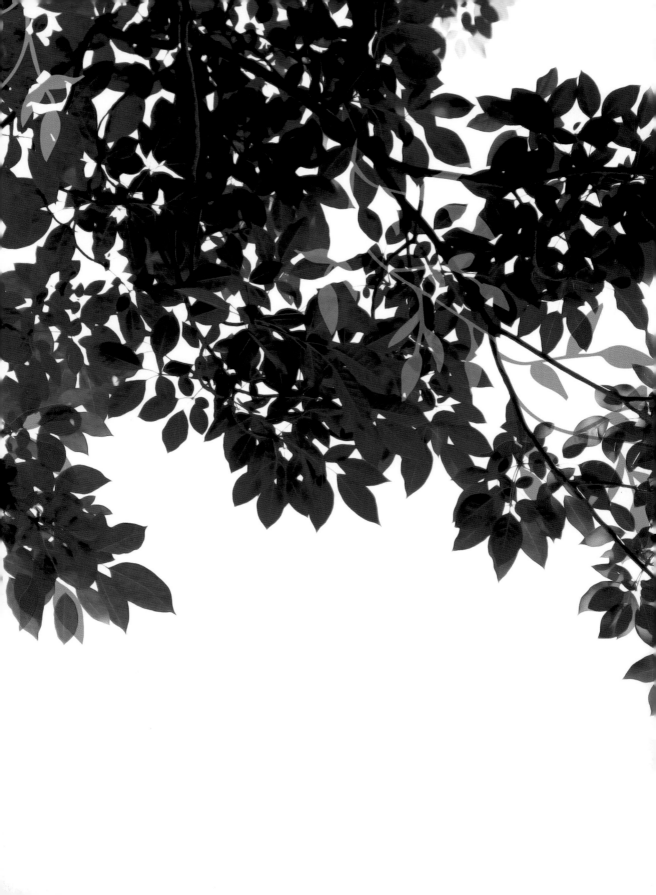

SIX

SKINCARE INGREDIENTS

the NEED-TO-KNOW INGREDIENTS

Deciphering the ingredients of beauty products can be like trying to understand a foreign language! Some plant names are unrecognisable. You may have read about retinol, hyaluronic acid, antioxidants and many of the latest 'wonder' ingredients, but ended up more confused. I love natural plant ingredients and taking a holistic approach, combined with a scientific one. To help demystify the more technical ingredients, I've sorted some of the fact from the fiction to help you make better choices.

I've been in the beauty industry for a long time and I still get confused by some of the ingredient lists on products – they can be baffling!

Antioxidants

As anti-ageing ingredients, antioxidants are proven to be some of the most effective. Not only do they combat free-radical damage, which is responsible for signs of premature ageing, but they also prevent and reverse sun damage. So they both repair and protect the skin. There are many different antioxidants and all have their own skin benefits. I like to take a combined approach to maximise results. Research has shown some of the most effective topical antioxidants to be vitamins A, C and E, beta-carotene, resveratrol and the mineral selenium.

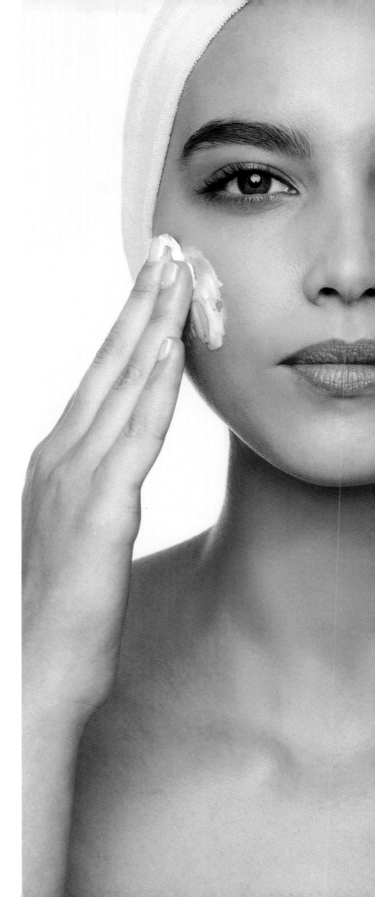

• VITAMIN C

This is a must when it comes to taking care of your skin. It boosts collagen production and skin plumpness, staves off UV damage, promotes skin healing and helps you achieve a brighter, more even-toned complexion. No wonder it's one of my skincare superheroes! Vitamin C is frequently labelled as ascorbic acid on product packaging. It's a great idea to apply a vitamin C serum and/or moisturiser to dry skin after cleansing, morning and night.

Top tips

1 Great to layer under your sunscreen as an extra antioxidant protection when outside.

2 Keep your vitamin C serum away from direct sunlight; it will break down and lose its effectiveness.

3 Vitamin C is even more effective when combined with vitamin E.

• VITAMIN E

An amazing skincare all-rounder, vitamin E is an oil-soluble antioxidant with high levels of plant oils. It's found naturally within the skin, but the amount falls when we're exposed to the sun and free radicals. Vitamin E helps to retain moisture, protect against environmental pollution, has anti-inflammatory properties and acts as a wound healer. It's also great for reducing redness, making it ideal for sensitive skins or if you're suffering from sunburn. You'll find it listed as tocopherol on ingredient labels.

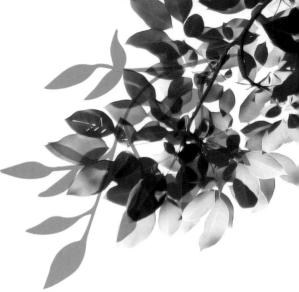

- **RETINOL**

Vitamin A itself is derived only from food (green leafy vegetables, fish, red and yellow vegetables) and cannot be made in the body on its own. It is created and stored in the liver.

Retinol is vitamin A in its whole form and it's one of the best ingredients for promoting skin regeneration. It forms part of a family of skincare ingredients called retinoids. It's a great 'cell-communicating' ingredient, which means it can send a message to almost any skin cell and tell it to behave like its younger, healthier self. Retinol is a mega-antioxidant, protecting your skin from free-radical damage and increasing both collagen production and cell turnover, helping your complexion look younger for longer. It's also great for fighting spots, reducing the appearance of pores and making pigmentation fade. Retinol turns into retinoic acid (also known as tretinoin), which speeds cell regeneration. Another ingredient you might see listed is retinyl palmitate, which is gentler and less irritating to the skin because it takes longer to be turned into retinoic acid.

Applying an SPF is non-negotiable if you have retinol in your skincare routine. And it shouldn't just be in your foundation – you need at least SPF 30.

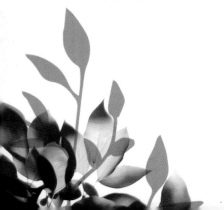

Retinol on prescription

Tretinoin: a prescription-strength pure retinoic acid that has an aggressive fast action, that's often prescribed for acne. Don't confuse it with your beauty product retinols because this is a much higher strength and can cause redness, peeling, itching and sensitivity.

Roaccutane: a vitamin-A derivative that's prescribed by doctors and taken in oral form if you're suffering from severe acne. It has numerous unpleasant side effects, and falling pregnant while on roaccutane is a big no. It thins and totally dries out the skin not just on the face and shouldn't be confused with topical cosmetics that contain small amounts of retinol. If you are taking Roaccutane, your home skincare regimen needs to contain extremely gentle products, an SPF 50 and you must still remain out of the sun. You should also avoid having facials or other treatments while taking it, and for six months after you complete the course.

Commonly asked questions

Q. Is retinol good for anti-ageing?
A. Yes! It brings visible benefits, but your skin needs a combination of ingredients to look and feel fantastic.

Q. Is retinol good for spots and large pores?
A. Yes. Although the size of your pores is determined by your genes, retinol can improve ones that have become enlarged or damaged. It tells lazy cells to wake up and function in a proper manner. In the case of enlarged pores, it reduces the 'sticky' build-up of cells and sebum (oil) inside them, so that they're less likely to get clogged. It also reduces the amount of sebum that your skin produces, so you have fewer blocked pores and fewer breakouts. So it's a win-win!

Q. Can I use retinol if I have sensitive skin?
A. Yes, unless you have super-sensitive skin or rosacea, but go steady when you start or it will cause redness, flaking and irritation. Begin with a low-strength retinol such as 0.3 per cent and apply it once or twice a week at night. Over a period of a month, slowly increase this to every other night, then every night. If at any point your skin becomes too sensitive, cut back until it rebalances again. Be aware that products contain different strengths and percentages, so always read the label.

Q. Can I use my other skincare while I'm using retinol?
A. Yes. Other products will prove essential when keeping the skin balanced and healthy. As your skin starts to look brighter and fresher, you might find that it is less in need of harsh cleansers and needs a little extra hydration.

Q. What about exfoliating?
A. Again yes. Exfoliators and retinol work well as a team! AHAs, BHAs and gritty exfoliants work from the surface of the skin down to remove dead cells. Retinol works at a deeper level within the dermis, so they support each other's actions. You may need to exfoliate less often than you did previously to avoid irritation. Listen to what your skin is telling you.

Q. When should I apply it?
A. You'll get the best out of your retinol if you apply it in the evening. It takes a number of hours to absorb fully, so it's best to allow it to do so when the skin is free from make-up or sunscreen. Let it work its magic on its own and save your vitamin C, hyaluronic acid or plant-based serum for the morning.

Q. How do I apply retinol?
A. Ideally it should be applied to cleansed and dried skin. Don't use it on your eyelids. Instead, apply it around the eyes, including over crow's feet, but not right up to your eyelashes as it will naturally travel inwards as it's absorbed.

Q. Can I use retinol if I'm pregnant?
A. It's best not to, but don't panic if you have. Ingesting large quantities of vitamin A in oral form has been linked to birth defects, but there's a huge difference between this and using a retinol skincare cream. The amounts are miniscule in comparison.

Q. Should I stop using retinol if I'm going on holiday?
A. I recommend stopping using retinol a week before you leave if you're going somewhere sunny. It's not about the extra heat or the sun making it less effective, more that new skin at the surface becomes vulnerable to sun damage when using retinol. There are so many other skin-nourishing products that would be better to pack – think hydrating toners, face oil, moisturiser and sunscreen! You can start applying retinol again two weeks after you return.

• PEPTIDES

Collagen boosters that stimulate the skin's stem cells. When collagen breaks down, it releases peptides. By applying a topical peptide, you're telling the skin to make new collagen. One of my favourites is copper peptide, which accelerates collagen production and also increases the skin's natural moisturising components. The result is firmer, more hydrated skin.

• ENZYMES

These are the gentlest form of skin peel, making them ideal for sensitive complexions. They're a lovely way of giving the skin a quick reboot, brightening and smoothing the surface. They work by gently eating up or dissolving dead skin and are generally labelled as natural fruit ingredients such as papaya, pineapple, mango, pumpkin or fig.

• ALPHA-HYDROXY ACIDS (AHAS)

Naturally occurring acids that induce an exfoliating action on the skin surface and help speed up cell turnover deeper down in the dermis. Put simply, AHAs are dead-skin blasters. If you picture your skin as a brick wall, AHAs work by loosening the cement in between the bricks/cells, allowing them to fall away more easily to reveal brighter, healthier, plumper new walls beneath. A number of studies have also shown AHAs to increase collagen production and dermal thickness, which softens the appearance of fine lines and gives the skin back its bounce. Because AHAs are usually in a water base, you should apply them to cleansed, dry skin, as oils will reduce their efficacy. Use them a maximum of three times a week if you have normal or oily skin. If you have sensitive skin, limit your use to once a week, or even once a month, if you find your skin is becoming irritated.

AHAs that you might find listed on a product ingredients label include:

Lactic acid: sour milk – offers good hydration. Of all the AHAs, lactic acid has some of the largest molecules, so it absorbs slowly. This means that it's less irritating on the skin and is unlikely to cause redness. It also has an amazing ability to increase your skin's own moisture levels.

Glycolic acid: a sugar – good for exfoliation. This has the smallest molecule size, so absorbs deep into the skin very quickly. It's been a popular ingredient for years, as it's a really effective exfoliating agent but it can feel quite irritating and some skins will turn pink after use!

Mandelic acid: made from bitter almonds – great for oily, problem skin as it has antibacterial properties.

Citric acid: found in lemons – good for lightening pigmented areas.

Azelaic acid: made from apples – good for breakouts.

Kojic acid: From mushrooms – again, great for pigmented areas.

A word of warning!
If you're using AHAs or have recently had a professional peel treatment, you must, must, must wear an SPF during the day. AHAs are exfoliating agents that work to remove the top layer of skin cells, so your skin quickly becomes more susceptible to sun damage.

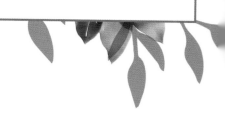

• BETA-HYDROXY ACIDS (BHAS)

BHAs clean out the inside of pores, which makes them especially good for acne and spot-prone skin. They're similar to AHAs, but whereas most AHAs will increase hydration, BHAs can have a drying effect. Unlike AHAs, BHAs won't make your skin more susceptible to sun damage. The most common BHA found in skincare is salicylic acid, a man-made ingredient derived from aspirin that has both anti-inflammatory and antibacterial properties.

• HYALURONIC ACID

This isn't actually an acid, it's a polysaccharide – basically a very large sugar. It's found naturally within our bodies, 50 per cent of it within our skin, and its highest concentration is inside the eyes and joints. It holds moisture in the spaces between the cells of our skin, helping it to stay plump. Babies' skin contains very high levels – it really is the source of 'baby soft' skin! It's one of the few skincare ingredients that will bring fast, visible benefits to all skin types. As we age, the levels in our skin begin to drop, most noticeably from forty onwards. The good news is that we can counteract this fall with the right products. It's often found in serum form and is derived from many sources, some plant and some animal. I like to apply it after cleansing and before moisturising – or mix it with another serum. It's great to soothe and rehydrate skin after exfoliating or having a professional peel and is safe to be used morning and night.

• TOPICAL PROBIOTICS

Many of us associate probiotics with yogurts that increase our so-called 'friendly bacteria' and boost our digestive health. We know they're good for our gut, but research shows that they can also benefit the skin. They're great for maintaining the natural pH balance of skin, making it healthier and more resilient to both intrinsic and extrinsic damage. Particular strains of bacteria have different benefits, such as helping to combat free-radical damage, reducing inflammation, increasing collagen production, acting as a natural moisturising factor and generally preventing the signs of ageing.

As discussed in chapter eight, maintaining the acidic environment of the skin surface is vital as it discourages bacterial growth and helps provide an effective moisture barrier. A recent study reported that the use of a fermented milk product containing lactic acid bacteria could also improve the structure of the skin's collagen. As a result, the researchers suggested using fermented milk on damaged skin to strengthen its collagen and repair process.

• STEM CELLS

In the skincare industry it's usually plant stem cells rather than human ones that are used. A handful of lesser-known brands use human stem-cell extracts but this would be clearly stated. Most cells have a specific purpose – if it's a brain cell that's what it will always be – but stem cells have the ability to adapt according to their surroundings into various types of cells. They are able to renew, replace and repair damaged cells. So in theory a stem cell within the skin would regenerate as a new skin cell.

Plant stem cells are extracts of cells rather than complete cells. Research has shown them to be a highly effective means of supporting the skin, because they act in a similar way of being impacted by their surroundings. I like to think of them as the superfoods of your skincare routine.

• HYDRAQUINONE

While this isn't an ingredient I'd generally recommend, it deserves a mention. Over-the-counter products containing hydroquinone have been linked with skin cancer and have been banned in several countries. As a bleaching agent, however, it has been used in the treatment of pigmentation. In my experience, while it will remove the pigmentation, as soon as you stop using the product, the problem will return – and often becomes worse. It's a complete no-no in the sun as it leaches away the skin's natural UV protectant factors and it mustn't be used in conjunction with salicylic acid or retinol. It should also never be used if you're pregnant or breastfeeding.

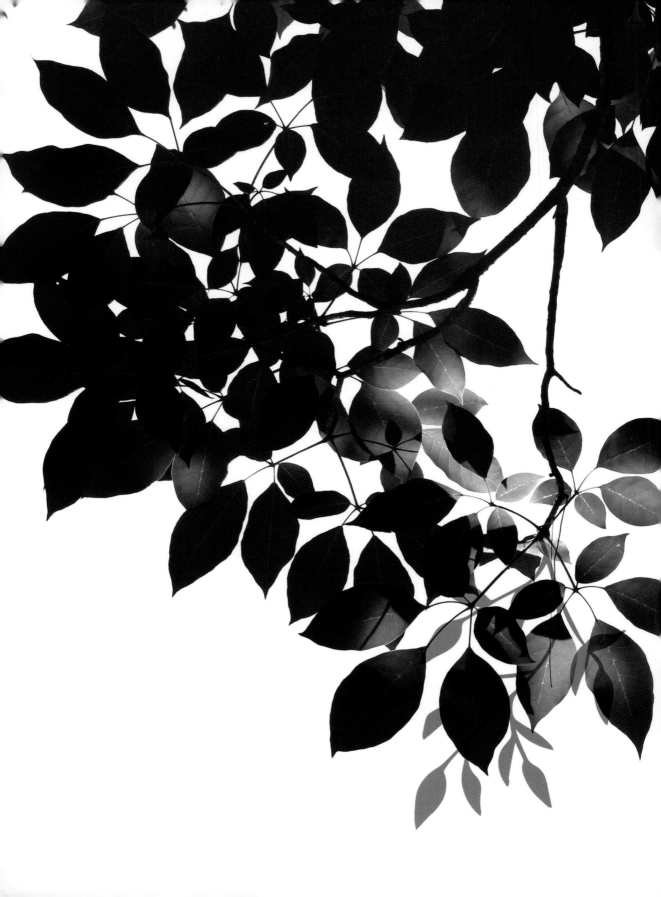

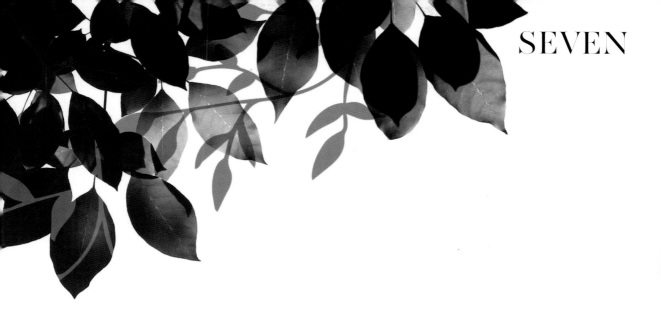

SEVEN

SKIN FITNESS

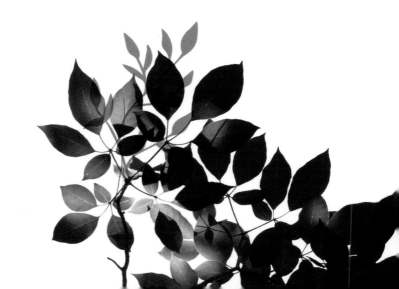

WHAT *your* FACE *is* TELLING YOU

> " Our faces reveal so many emotions. You can look at someone and immediately see whether they're sad, stressed, angry or happy.

At the end of a long day, other than the joy of seeing my children, very little beats the feeling of giving myself a face massage. Or a lazy pyjama Sunday morning face massage, with breakfast and papers in bed. I see and feel stress removed from my face. This chapter is all about giving you the confidence to use the power of your hands to rejuvenate your complexion – and your mind. These techniques are based on traditional therapies that are known for their ability to contribute to a healthy, glowing, vibrant complexion. Our faces reveal so many emotions. You can look at someone and immediately see whether they're sad, stressed, angry or happy and it's the muscles underlying the skin which form these different expressions. Like all muscles, they are susceptible to gravity and the wear and tear of age, so we need to keep them healthy.

According to Traditional Chinese Medicine (TCM), specific areas of the face relate to different internal organs and systems. This means that any skin concerns present on areas of the face – including breakouts, redness, dry patches, swelling and deep wrinkles – may be caused by deeper underlying issues or imbalances connected with organs and systems inside the body. The benefits of TCM have been well documented over thousands of years. It's not as simple as a breakout in a particular area indicating a specific problem with an organ.

The lower cheeks, for example, relate to the lung meridian, but if you suffer from recurring spots there, it doesn't necessarily mean that you have a problem with your respiratory system. The lung meridian has an emotional association and the breakouts may be caused by grief, anxiety, lack of self-esteem or depleted energy levels. If home products don't seem to be doing the trick, you may find TCM helps you to find the root cause of your problem. It is all about restoring balance and promoting the free flow of energy known as chi. Chi is the life force that travels through channels known as meridians.

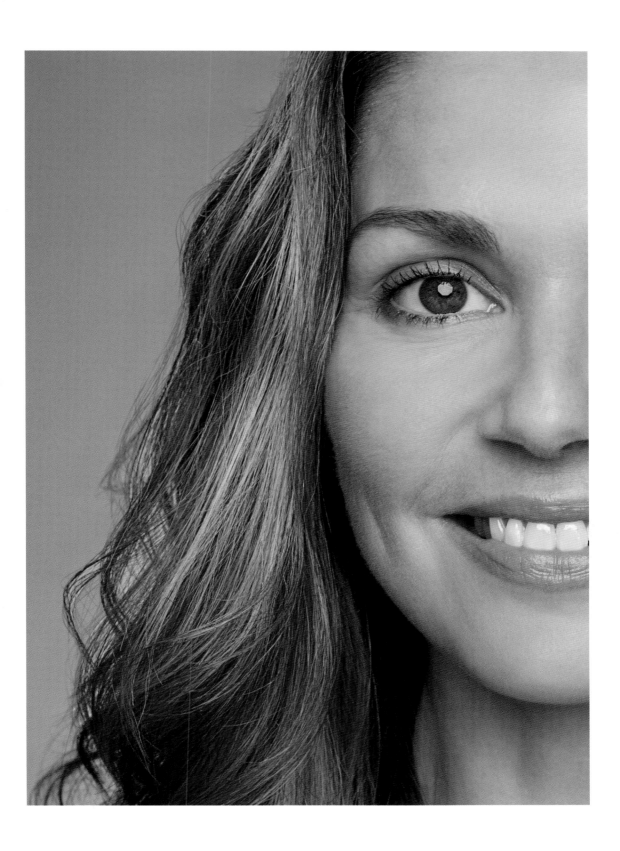

What *your* skin is telling you

LUNG
- Grief, stress or sad news.
- A low immune system. Try boosting with supplements.
- Skin issues such as eczema.
- Sweating too much can also indicate an imbalance within this meridian.

LIVER
- Anger, moodiness, irritability, irregular periods, PMS and general menstrual health.
- Constipation.
- A problem with the whole eye area; flare-ups of eczema are not uncommon around and on eyelids when you are angry/frustrated. Interestingly, the vertical lines between the eyebrows that we get from frowning are often referred to as 'liver lines'.
- Excess toxins, too much fatty food, alcohol, dairy. Clean up your diet by drinking green juice, milk thistle, filtered water.

HEART
- The heart is all about joy; any emotion associated with a lack of happiness and emotional stress can show up as redness in this area. Cut back on red meat and increase your omega oils.

SPLEEN AND STOMACH
- Worry, digestive issues, irritable bowel syndrome (IBS), constipation, over-working, adrenal fatigue, feeling generally run down.
- Puffiness may be due to an allergy and sluggish digestion. Increase your gut hydration and fibre intake.

KIDNEY
- Fear, feeling isolated, fertility issues, polycystic ovary syndrome (PCOS), urinary issues and problems relating to the kidneys may result in puffiness and water retention, which will be exacerbated by lack of sleep and too much caffeine, sugar and salt. Drink and eat lots of water and support your lymphatic system with regular Epsom salt baths and body brushing.

GALLBLADDER
- Lack of courage and indecision and issues linked to the liver. Can indicate a diet too high in fatty, over-processed foods.

COLON
- Blackheads and spots may be due to a sluggish digestive system and constipation. On an emotional level, worry and over thinking can affect the digestion.

FOREHEAD
- General digestive issues, bad diet, too much sugar, bad fats, excess rich foods and not enough water. Clear out your diet and increase your water intake.
- When there is an internal food allergy I often see small, under-the-skin pimples spread across this whole area.

CHIN AND JAW
- Connected to the hormonal system, with the ovaries positioned either side of the mouth on the chin. Often you may break out on one side, which may indicate on which side you are ovulating.
- White spots on the chin, blotchy patches or a red chin can indicate too much sugar and gut candida.
- Spots to the side of the chin can also be related to the colon.

Feelings and emotions are part of being human. In chapter two I described how stress can affect our skin in ways you may not have thought of. In Chinese medicine, balancing our emotions is considered just as important as balancing our food and lifestyle. According to TCM, if you break out in the same area again and again, or deeper wrinkles appear in a specific area, the cause may be an emotional imbalance that diet and products alone can't budge.

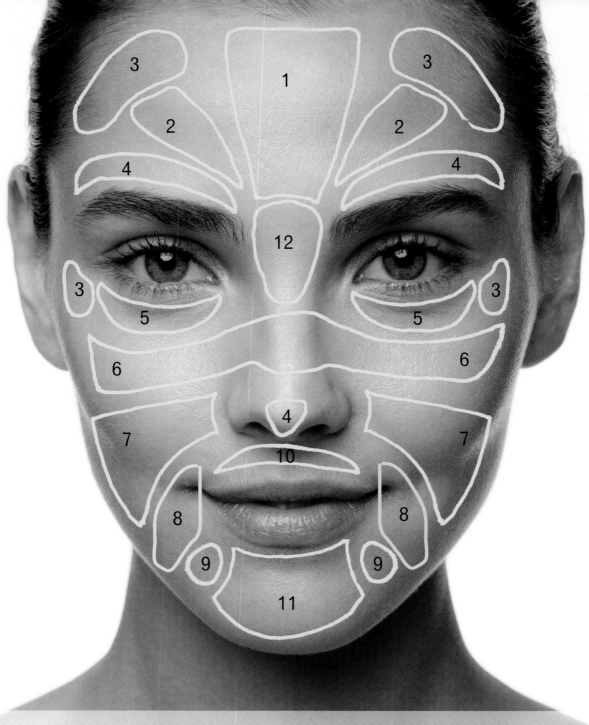

1. SMALL INTESTINE
2. BLADDER
3. GALLBLADDER
4. HEART
5. KIDNEYS
6. STOMACH/SPLEEN/PANCREAS
7. LUNGS
8. COLONS
9. OVARIES
10. SMALL INTESTINE/HEART
11. HORMONES/KIDNEYS/ENDOCRYNE
12. LIVER

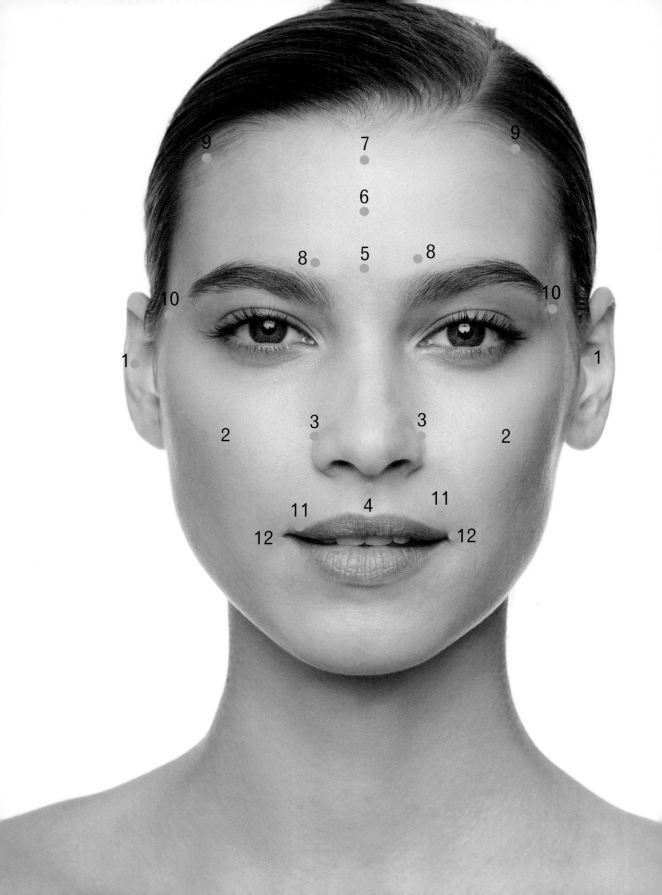

Facial acupressure

Acupressure follows the same principles as acupuncture, except it uses fingers rather than needles. A treatment by a trained therapist will be on a different level, but you can do it at home on a daily basis and instantly see visible results. It is deeply calming, and I love including it in my night-time skincare routine. The technique involves stimulating the internal organs via chi channels (meridians) to restore organ balance and reach the root cause of many skin concerns. Use your thumb or a finger to press firmly into each point. You can rotate or pump on each point or just hold for five to ten seconds while breathing really deeply and slowly. Don't worry about finding the exact point: you'll be stimulating local nerves and tissues even if you're not directly on the spot.

THE BENEFITS

- Improves circulation, releases tension within muscles and frees the flow of energy and blood. As most of these meridians begin and end on the face, you stimulate other areas of the body as well.

- Promotes blood flow to the skin surface, meaning more nutrients can reach the skin cells.

- Reduces muscle fatigue and increases elasticity, helping to reduce sagging and wrinkle formation.

- Stimulates the production of collagen, softening the skin and smoothing wrinkles.

- Soothes inflammation and supports inner detoxification channels.

---

1. Regulates all body functions, supports kidneys, eyes, mouth, nose, adrenal glands, stomach. Relaxes the nervous system, balances blood pressure, supports the immune system, aids digestion.
2. Supports lungs and heart, aids relaxation, facial paralysis and swelling, insomnia, sinusitis, sore eyes.
3. Lungs, liver, heart, stomach, spleen. Stimulates endorphins, soothes pain, anti-inflammatory.
4. Heart, lungs, nose, liver, stomach, colon. Increases blood flow and energy.

5. The 'Third Eye', between the brows. Stimulates the pituitary gland, supporting hormonal balance. Press and hold the point for 60 seconds daily. Relaxes, soothes jaw pain, insomnia, worry.
6. Throat, eyes, neck, forehead. Promotes concentration and soothes issues relating to the head, including jaw pain, insomnia, worry.
7. Forehead, eyes, liver, pituitary gland. Good for regulating hormones. Clears the mind.

8. Sinuses, eyes, heart. Relaxes the nervous system and promotes sleep. Soothes pain, relaxes muscles.
9. Gallbladder, spleen. Calms the nervous system, insomnia, aids general skin problems.
10. Eye pain, eye problems, brightens eyes, thyroid, insomnia.
11. Pancreas, hormones. Promotes healthy digestion.
12. Supports adrenal glands, kidneys. Good anti-inflammatory point.

The power of touch

All natural face-lifting methods have one thing in common: they rely on specific, repetitive movements to stimulate blood flow, remove toxins and release tension. Improved muscle tone supports the skin better, lifting and softening your facial contours, smoothing lines and wrinkles and boosting the overall health of your skin. Not to mention calming the mind.

The benefits of face massage

- It's a drug-free, non-invasive way of benefiting your skin

- Increases circulation, allowing the body to pump more oxygen and nutrients into tissues, working beyond the face

- Stimulates the flow of lymph, the body's natural defence system, helping to reduce puffiness and speed up general detoxification of the skin

- Gives an instant glow and lift

- Speeds skin cell turnover

The best time to perform a face massage depends on your lifestyle. It might be in the evening after you've removed your make-up. Or in the morning before you cleanse. I keep an oil both in the shower and by the bath so I can massage my face either in the morning or the evening and don't need to worry about washing off any excess oil.

BEFORE YOU START: This is best avoided if you have super-sensitive skin, rosacea, acne, or if you've spent too long in the sun.

WHAT TO MASSAGE WITH: Ideally a plant-based oil (not a mineral oil or paraffin liquid, as these will just coat your skin like cling film and block your pores) such as:

- **Coconut oil:** incredibly nourishing and super-hydrating, so particularly good for dry skin. It contains antioxidants, is anti-inflammatory and antibacterial. It's also rich in high saturated fatty acids, which means it's solid at room temperature – so there won't be spillages if you use it at night before climbing into bed.

- **Argan oil:** loved by the hair and beauty industry, it has high levels of vitamin E and sterols, which make it soothing and good for healing skin and reducing inflammation.

- **Rosehip seed oil:** light yet nourishing, it's full of vitamins, antioxidants and EFAs that are known to correct dark spots, hydrate, reduce fine lines and support scar healing.

- **Sea buckthorn oil:** neither too oily nor too light, it contains high levels of vitamins B and C, as well as omegas 7 and 9. It's great for cell regeneration and skin healing. Supposedly good for fighting fungal infections, which is why it's used in many nail treatments.

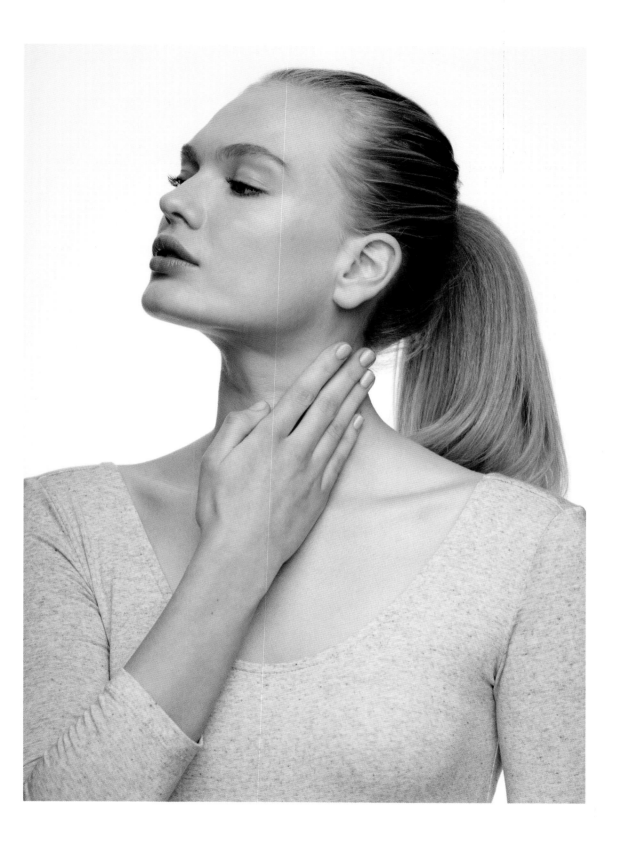

Lifting face massage: the routine

Warm half a teaspoon of oil in your palms, then apply in a prayer movement to your face, neck and décolletage.

---

1. Using the right hand make big, downward circles on the left side of the neck. Repeat on the other side using the other hand.

2. Using both hands together, massage both sides of the neck at the same time.

3. Make scissor shapes with your middle and index fingers. Place the index finger behind the ear and the middle in front. Push your hands back and forth either side of the ears and along the jaw – this supports the lymph and drainage.

4. Hold your hands out in front of your face with your fingers splayed, place your thumbs under your chin, push and drain under your jaw from the chin to the ears.

5. Keep your thumbs under your chin and make a pinch with the sides of the index fingers. Pinch and push out along the jaw. Pressing firmly, make circular moves around the mouth.

6. Concentrating on one side of the face, use alternate hands to push up, lifting the cheek. Repeat on the other side.

7. Make a fist with both hands and press your knuckles into the cheeks, just under the cheekbone. Look down to increase pressure, hold for the count of five, then glide your knuckles out to the sides. Knuckle massage your whole cheek area.

8. Using all your fingers, push up just under the brow and glide outwards.

9. Using the finger pads of both hands, firmly stretch crow's feet. Hold each stretch for five seconds.

10. Using your middle and index fingers, stretch and hold the frown lines.

11. Still on the frown lines, firmly make a criss-cross movement. Continue criss-crossing across the whole of the forehead. Change the direction of your fingers and zig-zag up and down over the forehead.

12. Calm everything down with some gentle smoothing outward 'prayers'. Finish by gliding alternate hands in the direction of the lymph out from under the chin to the ear and drain down the neck. Repeat on the other side.

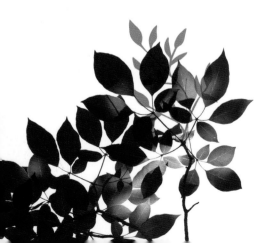

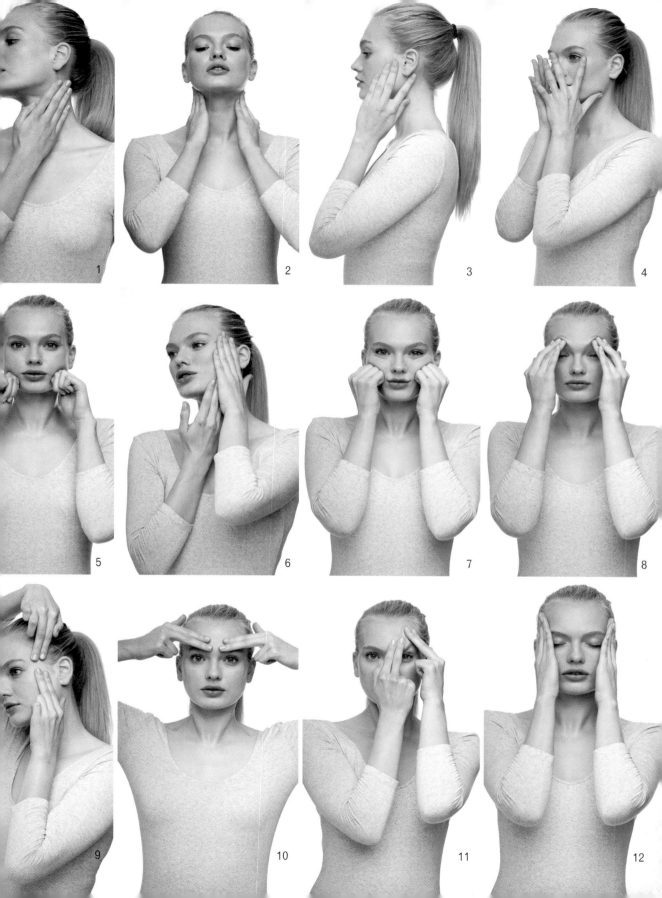

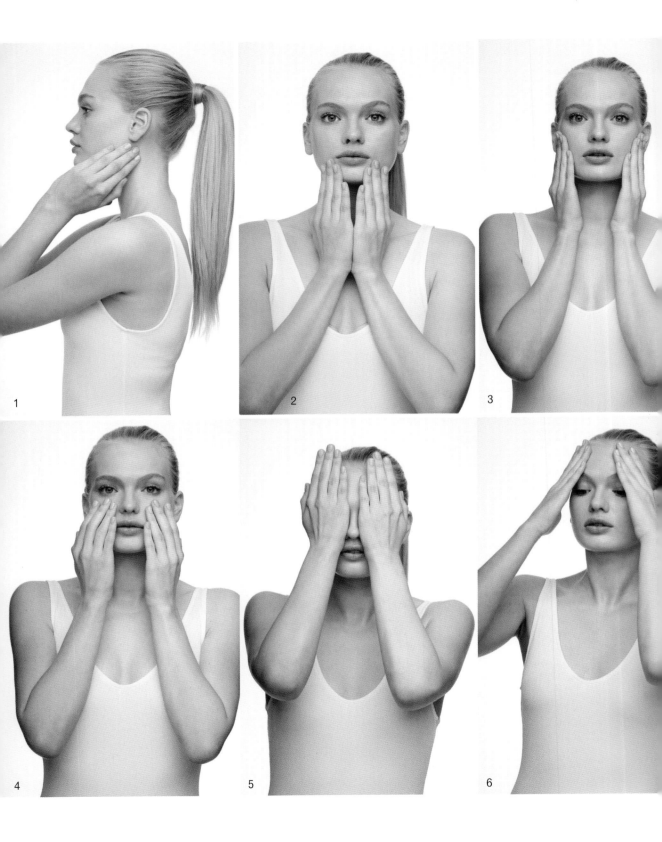

Soothing face massage to beat puffiness

Sensitive skins and those with acne and rosacea need a massage that works with the lymphatic system. For best results, it should be done at least twice a week.

THE BENEFITS

- Disperses fluid and puffiness caused by illness, overindulgence, surgery or cosmetic treatments
- Calms redness, inflammation, swelling and sensitivity
- Helps ease sinusitis
- Reduces the appearance of scar tissue

The lymphatic system is known as the secondary circulatory system but, unlike the heart, it doesn't have a pump to make it flow. Essentially, it's a filtering system to remove toxins. It relies upon breathing, muscular movement and peristalsis. Lymph nodes are located all around the body. They produce white blood cells that defend the body against infection, bacteria and poisons. Encouraging the flow of lymph is vital to reducing the visible effects of inflammation and to supporting the healing process.

THE ROUTINE

A gentle, rhythmical massage performed with a down-and-out movement, without any oil or cream. If you press too hard it will be less effective, so you need a super-soft touch. Ideally wear a low-cut top, tie your hair back, cleanse your skin and wash your hands.

1. With fingers together facing backwards, place your hands on your neck with your little fingers just beneath your earlobes. Make a downward pumping movement, then allow the skin to spring back. Keeping your hands in the same position, change to a forward pumping movement.

2. Place the pads of your fingers on your chin, and pump downwards. Move your hands out across your jaw and repeat.

3. Place your hands flat on the sides of your face, just in front of your ears. Your index finger should be just touching your ear. Make an outward pumping movement, gently stretching the sides of the mouth. Place the pads of your fingers above your top lip and repeat this pumping action. Move your hands back to your cheeks, and pump downwards.

4. Place your finger pads just below your eyes and, very, very gently, make the pumping action, downwards.

5. Place the palms of your hands over your eyes and very gently repeat this pumping action.

6. Place flat hands in the middle of your forehead and, using the full length of your fingers, pump downwards. Move your hands out slightly and repeat. Gently glide your hands out across the forehead, across the cheeks, down the neck and finish with your hands in an open fan.

Repeat each move seven times. The routine can take a bit of practice but it will quickly come quite naturally.

Facial yoga

This anti-ageing technique has been practised through the centuries by many a famous face dating as far back as Cleopatra. Facial yoga – or facial fitness – helps to keep facial muscles firm, toned and healthy, in much the same way as traditional yoga improves the muscles of the body. The most effective way to achieve a balanced body is to combine a variety of exercise styles. The same is true of the face.

THE BENEFITS

- Radiance
- Firmer facial contours
- Inner confidence
- Bright eyes
- A happy face – with a relaxed expression

DOES IT WORK?

With practice and patience, yes. It's about learning to isolate the muscles, something that takes time to learn. The muscles that control our facial expressions are small, delicate and move constantly throughout the day. As we age and the skin's collagen and elastin production slows, it becomes less able to withstand the pull of gravity, so we develop lines and sagging. By strengthening the underlying structure, we can help the skin to look its best for longer. If you combine home facial yoga with professional treatments such as microcurrent (see page 178), which work facial muscles to boost cell energy, you'll really see results.

THE ROUTINES

Start by doing them in front of a mirror. Remember to relax your face – even when doing yoga for the body, we can have a furrowed brow or clenched jaw as we try to hold a pose.

1. Jaw and side of face

Open your mouth and chew. Using firm finger pressure massage 'finger circles' across the jaw and cheek area to release the jaw while you continue to chew.
Benefit: eases jaw and facial tension, particularly for those who grind their teeth.

2. 'The face-lifter'

Sit up straight, relax your shoulders and hold your left arm out to the side about 45 degrees away from your body. Take the right arm straight up in the air towards the ceiling. Bend this arm over your head to make contact with the left side of the face. Relax your shoulders, breathe, then, using your right hand, begin to stretch the head away. You should feel a stretch in the left side of your face and neck. Repeat on the other side.
Benefit: lifts the side of the face and reduces facial tension.

3. 'The Big O'

Pull your lips tightly over your teeth and smile. Close your eyes firmly without scrunching. Take this one step further by massaging with a finger (or fingers), making small circles around the chin and top lip.
Benefit: smooths lip lines, lifts and firms cheeks.

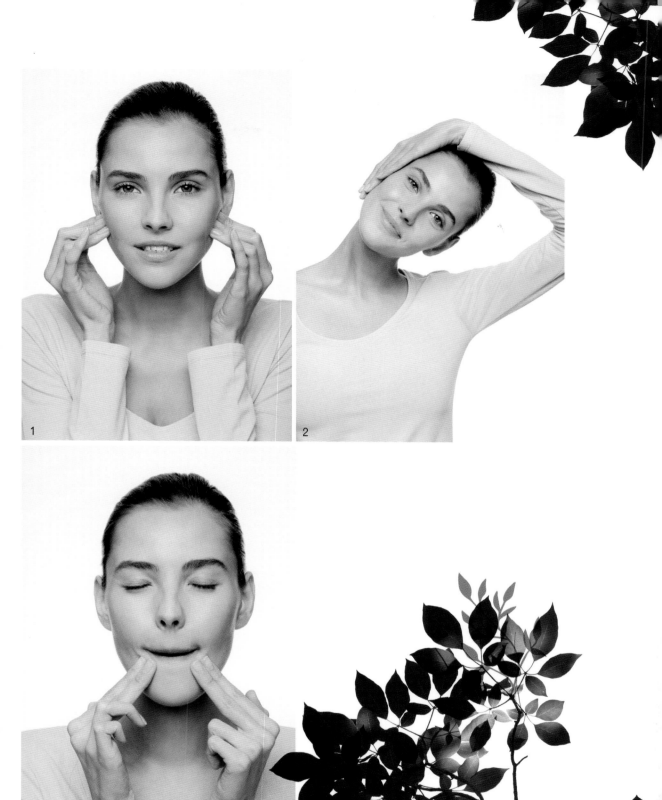

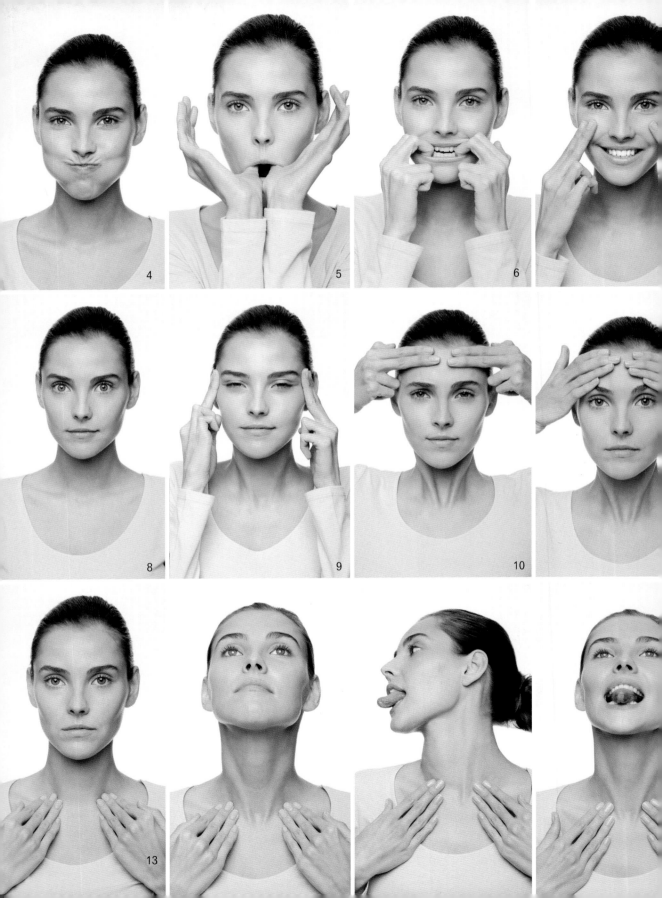

4

5

6

8

9

10

13

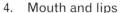

4.   Mouth and lips

'Puffer fish' Fill your cheeks and the area around the mouth with air. Swap air from cheek to cheek, holding for five seconds each time, then blow out with a bumble bee lip vibration.
Benefit: softens the nasolabial lines, smooths the appearance of the cheeks and plumps lips.

5.   Lip and line smoother

With wrists together, place your thumbs inside your mouth. Push out with your thumbs, then close your mouth firmly in an 'O' shape around your thumbs. Hold and release five times.
Benefit: softens lip lines, nasolabial lines and lost volume around the lips.

6.   Lower lip smoother

Place your middle and index fingers inside your lower lip. Purse your lips around them, hold and release as many times as you want.
Benefit: softens lines around the mouth and nasolabial lines.

7.   Apples of cheeks

Place the pads of your fingers on the apples of your cheeks, apply pressure and smile. Pulse ten times.
Benefit: keeps your cheeks perky and helps define cheekbones.

8.   Surprise eyes

Concentrate on holding your eyes open and not wrinkling your brow.
Benefit: a major brow smoother, it also works the muscles around the eyes.

9.   Crow's feet smoother

Place flat fingers by the sides of your eyes and support with tension. Blink without fully closing your eyes; feel the lower lid tighten.
Benefit: smooths lines all around the eyes.

10. Upper lid lift

Place your fingertips on each brow, lift slightly, but not too high. Hold and blink your eyes closed firmly, but without scrunching down.
Benefit: supports drooping eyelids and opens the eyes.

11. Forehead

Brow lift: Hold flat fingers across your brow, frown with pressure against the resistance, but not deep enough to cause frown lines.
Benefit: smoothes the forehead.

12. Upper brow lift

Place the sides of flat fingers in your hair line, lift, then frown against this pressure.
Benefit: lifts the entire frontalis forehead muscle.

13. Jowls and neck 'Slack attack'

I created this routine in response to clients' concerns about double chins and slackening of the lower face and neck area. These moves work perfectly as a home-care support alongside radiofrequency treatments to firm and tone (see page 178).

Place your fingertips just above the collarbone, apply a little pressure (enough to support the skin), look up, tilting your head backwards. You should feel the stretch in the front of the neck.

Flatten your tongue on the roof of your mouth. Hold and pulse your tongue against the roof of the mouth five times.

Stick out your tongue, first to the left, then to the middle and then to the right. Hold each position for five seconds.

Take your lower lip over your top lip and hold; turn to the left, turn to the right.

With your lower lip over your top lip, press your tongue to the roof of your mouth.

Turn your head to the side, look up, then put your tongue on the roof of your mouth and swallow.

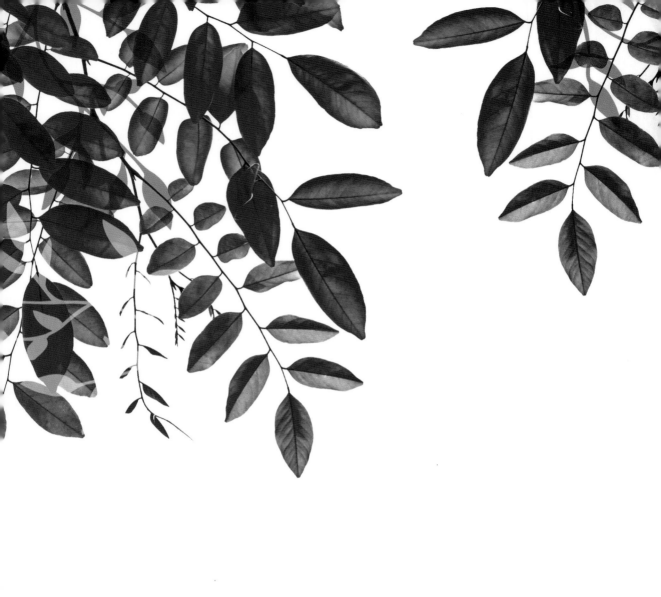

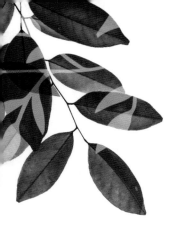

EIGHT

SKIN FOOD

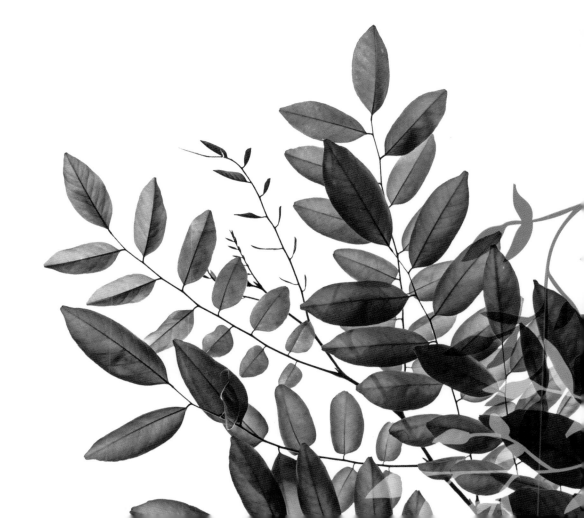

Not only do you need to provide your skin with the right nutrients, you also need to ensure that your body is absorbing them effectively. This is why maintaining good gut health alongside a balanced diet is important. Our modern-day diets can be incredibly unforgiving on our digestive systems. Sadly, the result is all too often inflammation, hormonal imbalances and even long-term illness. Inside the digestive tract, there are millions of bacteria – some friendly and some not so friendly! High levels of bad bacteria inhibit the body's ability to absorb the vitamins, minerals and other essential nutrients efficiently. As a result, the gut becomes inflamed – which is why the number of people with food intolerances is on the rise.

FOUR WAYS
to good GUT HEALTH

1. Increase your intake of foods containing a direct source of friendly bacteria.

2. Eat foods that feed the good bacteria to create a friendly environment.

3. Avoid foods that attract bad bacteria.

4. Take a multi-strain probiotic supplement.

DIRECT FOOD SOURCES OF FRIENDLY BACTERIA
Naturally fermented foods such as sauerkraut, kefir, kombucha, tempeh, fermented miso, kimchi and cultured yogurt. These are known as 'probiotic' foods.

FOOD SOURCES FOR FRIENDLY BACTERIA
This includes foods that contain certain types of fibre called inulin, fructo-oligosaccharides (FOS) and galacto-oligosaccharides (GOS). These can be found in green olives, green bananas, Jerusalem artichokes, asparagus, onions, leeks, shallots, garlic, spring onions and fennel. These are known as 'prebiotic' foods.

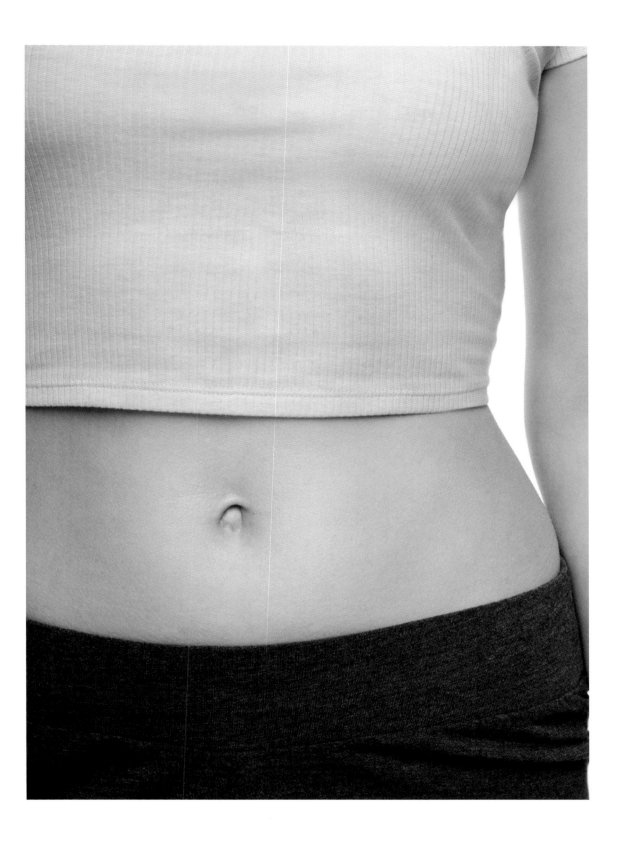

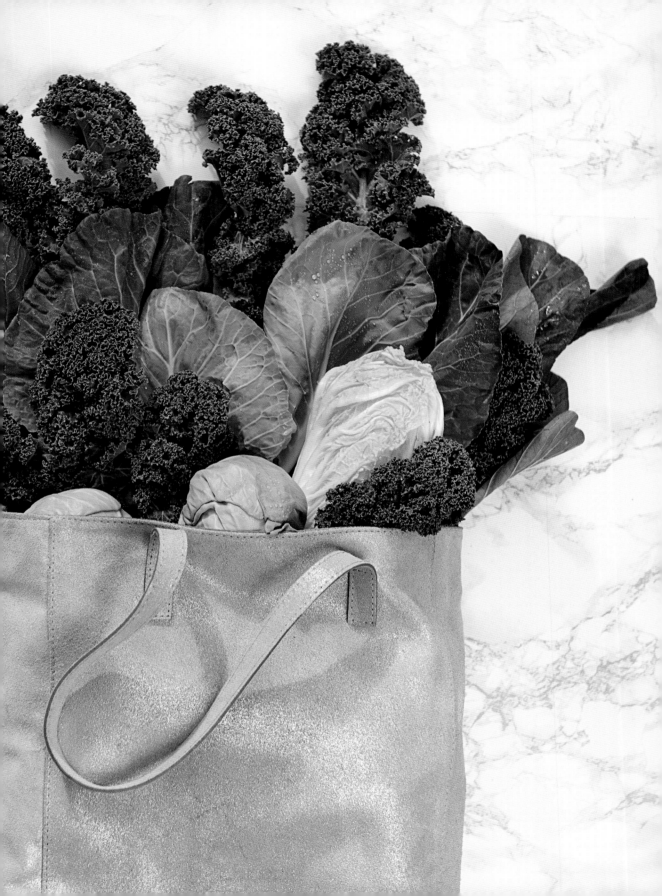

WHY THE LIVER IS IMPORTANT TO YOUR SKIN HEALTH

The health of the liver is vital to the vibrancy and clarity of the skin. Its role is to remove toxins such as pesticides from food, medication, pollution, alcohol and caffeine. It re-packages them so that they can be safely removed via the digestive system. It is also responsible for processing hormones, so if it's not functioning correctly, these hormones get re-circulated around the body. This is why the liver plays such a key role in adult acne, breakouts and problematic skin types.

A common reason why the liver becomes overloaded is constipation. When this happens, toxins get stuck in the gut and are re-routed back to the liver, so they end up being detoxified – twice! The best thing is to get the digestive system moving by increasing your intake of fibre and probiotic-rich foods. Anyone suffering from constipation should not attempt a liver detoxification programme.

Kick start your liver and begin each day with a cup of the following: hot water with lemon, turmeric and cayenne pepper or fresh ginger.

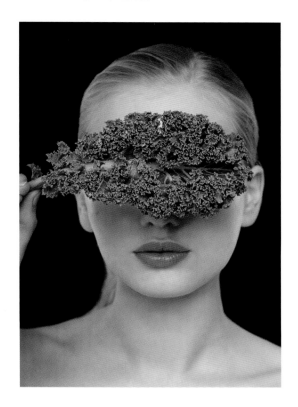

How to support the liver

When you are ready to start cleansing your liver, you can follow a few simple steps.

STEP 1. Cut down on anything that will aggravate your liver, such as alcohol, sugar, hydrogenated fats and caffeine.

STEP 2. Eat more 'clean foods' that help the liver break down toxins. This means cruciferous vegetables such as broccoli, cabbage and dark green leafy vegetables (watercress, spinach, rocket, kale and spring greens). Other foods or food groups that optimise liver health include berries, citrus fruits, fresh herbs and spices, especially turmeric.

STEP 3. Supplements such as milk thistle and chlorella help to restore liver function and act as an anti-inflammatory.

LET'S TALK ABOUT INFLAMMATION

A hot topic in skincare as research has progressed, inflammation not only speeds up the ageing process, it also aggravates skin conditions such as acne, rosacea, psoriasis and eczema. The digestive tract is a common place for inflammation to start – often with a food intolerance caused by an imbalance in the ratio of good to bad bacteria.

1 ANTI-INFLAMMATORY FOODS

Herbs and spices, especially ginger and turmeric, plus garlic. Healthy oils such as cold-pressed olive oil, coconut, flaxseed, avocado and hemp.

2 ANTIOXIDANT-RICH FOODS

Oily fish such as salmon, mackerel and sardines, as well as nuts and seeds.

3 SOURCES OF SOLUBLE AND INSOLUBLE FIBRE

These will help ensure that you have a bowel movement at least once a day. So increase your intake of apples, bananas, berries, oats, nuts and seeds (especially flaxseed and chia – accompanied by water).

4 FOODS TO AVOID

Anything that's high in saturated fats and white sugar such as white bread, sweets, fried food, ice cream, fruit juice from cartons, pasta, cream cheese, pizza, fizzy drinks, processed meat.

5 PROBIOTICS

We've already looked at the role probiotics play in restoring optimal microbial balance within the gut. There's also increasing interest in their use in treating inflammatory and allergic conditions.

6 ANTIOXIDANTS

Essential when it comes to supporting the ageing process, they help protect against free-radical damage, which can weaken the natural skin defences. There are both fat-soluble and water-soluble antioxidants, both of which should be consumed regularly through a wide variety of fresh fruit and vegetables. Fat-

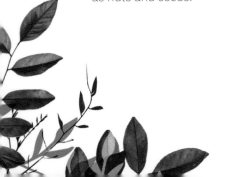

soluble antioxidants are best absorbed when you've eaten something containing good fats, so I combine them with a little olive or flaxseed oil.

7 VITAMIN C

Crucial for maintaining healthy skin with a good amount of elasticity, collagen and plumpness, vitamin C can be depleted by the presence of sunlight within the skin, which is another excellent reason to stay in the shade or at the very least, apply SPF on a daily basis. It's worth noting that the body can't store or manufacture vitamin C, so we need to make sure our daily diet includes plenty.

TOP FOODS: Watercress, grapefruit, red pepper, kale, kiwi, broccoli.

8 VITAMIN A

A fat-soluble antioxidant often used in skincare. There are two forms: retinol and beta-carotene, both of which can be found in food. Retinol is in meat, liver, eggs and some cheeses; beta-carotene can be obtained from red, orange and yellow fruit and vegetables. Beta-carotene gets converted into vitamin A when the body requires it. When levels are low, our skin can become dry and flaky because one of its primary functions is to regulate the shedding of the upper layer of skin cells to help keep the surface smooth.

Vitamin A also helps slow down cell ageing and is a must for those with acne or problematic skin as it helps prevent oil from building up.

TOP FOODS: 150g kale contains around 80 per cent of your recommended daily requirement of vitamin A. I love to bake it in the oven with some olive oil and salt to make delicious kale crisps. Most other leafy greens are also very high in vitamin A, as are orange fruit and vegetables such as apricots, sweet potatoes and carrots.

9 VITAMIN B

This is a group of vitamins that is underestimated when it comes to understanding its impact on our skin's health. A deficiency in B vitamins can cause cracks to form at the corners of the mouth, or the skin around the nose to become red and greasy. A very pale complexion can be a symptom of a lack of vitamin B12. Both B2 and B5 reduce facial oiliness and restore your skin's natural glow. B3 (niacin) plays a key role in maintaining the skin's barrier protection, keeping moisture in and irritants out. It's been known to be helpful in the treatment of sensitive skins and rosacea, and help minimise dark spots. B2 (riboflavin) is also essential for healthy cell growth and repair, so accelerates healing, reduces scarring and soothes eczema.

TOP FOODS: eggs, poultry, fish, mushrooms, beans, lentils, quinoa, wholemeal rice, seeds, oats, watermelons plus a variety of vegetables.

10 VITAMIN E

This is a fat-soluble vitamin found mainly in foods with a natural fat content. Vitamin E is one of the most well-known beneficial skin nutrients as it moves easily into fatty layers of tissue to protect our collagen and prevent free-radical damage.

TOP FOODS: avocado, sesame seeds, sunflower seeds, nuts, olives and olive oil.

11 COENZYME Q10

This helps to make a fuel known as adenosine triphosphate (ATP) for your body to use. ATP is the powerhouse of our cells and without it the ageing process accelerates rapidly. It's also a powerful antioxidant that has been shown to improve elasticity. When you combine coenzyme Q10 with other antioxidants, such as vitamins C, E and selenium, it supercharges the energising, skin-renewal effect.

TOP COENZYME FOODS: oily fish, organ meats and whole grains, peanuts, spinach, cauliflower and broccoli.

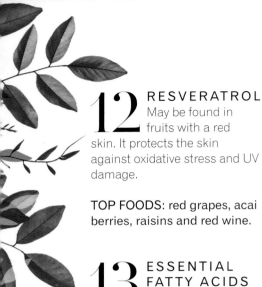

12 RESVERATROL
May be found in fruits with a red skin. It protects the skin against oxidative stress and UV damage.

TOP FOODS: red grapes, acai berries, raisins and red wine.

13 ESSENTIAL FATTY ACIDS (EFAS)
The body can't manufacture EFAs – so we have to obtain them from the foods we eat. They are vital if we're to have healthy skin as they hold potent anti-inflammatory powers, so reduce sensitivity whilst simultaneously plumping and hydrating it. They really are skin superstars! There are two main types: omega-3 and omega-6; which need to be balanced. Too much omega-6 will upset your hormonal balance.

TOP OMEGA-3 FOODS: flaxseed, tuna, mackerel and salmon.

TOP OMEGA-6 FOODS: sunflower and hemp seeds.

14 MINERALS
Vitamins are organic and found in living things – plants and animals – whereas minerals are inorganic and found in liquids and soil. They're absorbed by plants or eaten by animals.The body doesn't need all minerals but some are essential.

15 ZINC
This is a trace mineral, which means we only need small amounts of it. From regulating our hormones to supporting our immune system, zinc is involved in many processes inside the body. It's commonly used in the treatment of skin complaints as it helps to stimulate healing and has a direct effect on the sebaceous glands, working to rebalance our complexion if it's too oily or too dry.

TOP FOODS: pumpkins and their seeds, sweet potato, lentils and other legumes, quinoa and shellfish.

16 SELENIUM
Another trace mineral, we need it to produce other antioxidants that protect skin cells and collagen fibres. It's also essential for those with acne and inflamed skin as it has amazing calming properties.

TOP FOODS: Brazil nuts are super-high in selenium. Just four to five a day can provide all your skin needs to help slow down the ageing process. Chicken is another rich source.

17 MAGNESIUM
According to one study, skin cells that are grown without magnesium are twice as likely to suffer attacks from free radicals. Low levels of magnesium will have a detrimental impact on skin elasticity and moisture levels by depleting its fatty acid content. Magnesium is essential for reducing inflammation, so is great to combat a wide array of troublesome skin conditions such as acne, eczema and premature skin ageing.

TOP FOODS: green leafy vegetables, bananas, avocado, brown rice, nuts and seeds, dark chocolate and dried figs.

18 CALCIUM
It's not just dairy products that contain calcium. There are many other rich sources. Calcium helps to control how often skin cells divide and maintains the integrity of the skin's natural protective barrier. The more flexible the skin barrier is, the easier it is for substances to pass into and out of our cells. So calcium helps waste products be removed and vital nutrients enter the cell.

Without adequate calcium, we develop dry, flaky skin that's itchy and ages prematurely.

TOP FOODS: dark green leafy vegetables, nuts, seeds, figs and salmon.

19 IRON
Iron promotes oxygenation of the blood, supports a

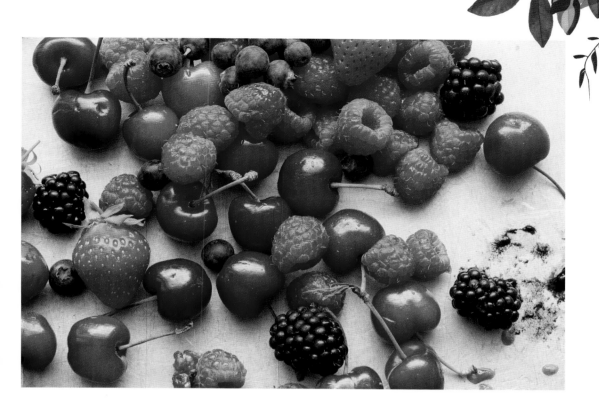

healthy immune system and accelerates wound healing. If you suffer from a very dull complexion or frequent breakouts, it will help ensure that enough fresh blood flows to the skin surface to speed it on its way back to optimum health.

TOP FOODS: dried apricots, figs, chickpeas, lentils and pumpkin seeds.

20 SILICA

This gives our hair, bones and nails their strength. If we don't have enough of it, our skin becomes droopy, itchy and dry. Silica has an extraordinary ability to bind up to 300 times its own weight in water, so is also essential for maintaining skin moisture levels and plumpness.

TOP FOODS: cucumber, rhubarb and strawberries (rhubarb stewed with strawberries and cinnamon, served with coconut yogurt or chia pudding is one of my all-time favourite breakfasts).

21 LYCOPENE

This is one of the best free-radical scavengers – even more so than vitamin A! It streamlines the way our skin cells communicate with one another and how fast they're able to reproduce. This means collagen is able to repair itself more efficiently – so we get fewer wrinkles. Lycopene also increases your skin's built-in sun protection factor, giving it a natural SPF of around 3 – before you've even applied sunscreen.

TOP FOODS: tomatoes and watermelon, papaya, guava.

22 VITAMIN K

Plays an important role in blood clotting, working to reduce dark under-eye circles by strengthening capillary walls.

TOP FOODS: kale, basil, spring onions, Brussels sprouts, asparagus, chili powder.

my favourite skin-loving superfoods

Adding superfoods to my daily diet – mixed into smoothies, cereals or home baking – is an easy way of making sure my family and I are getting enough good nutrients. The children are blissfully unaware that the cool-looking green powder is so amazing for their health!

- **FLAXSEED AND CHIA** both contain omega-3 fatty acids, which help plump the skin and reduce redness and inflammation. They're real all-rounders!

- **ACAI** is a berry that originates from Brazil and is well known for its potent antioxidant properties. It's therefore perfect for including in skincare programmes, as it supports overall skin health and prevents our collagen being broken down.

- **SPIRULINA** is a blue-green microscopic plant that has been around for billions of years. It contains a high vegan protein content of about 60 to 70 per cent and is very bioavailable, which means it's easily absorbed by the body. Protein acts as the building blocks of healthy skin turnover and regeneration.

- **CHLORELLA** is a microalgae that contains a high concentration of chlorophyll. It's high in zinc and vitamin B2, which help promote clear and radiant skin and also assists detoxification. A body with a lower toxic load is a body with fewer skin issues!

- **BAOBAB** is the fruit taken from the baobab tree and often comes in powdered form. It contains more vitamin C than oranges, as well as minerals such as calcium, potassium and magnesium, which are all great for supporting collagen production and alkalising the body.

- **SUPER CACAO** is one of those 'wow' ingredients, as it contains key nutrients that support your whole body. It protects, repairs and prevents cell damage. With such a high level of cacao flavonols it benefits your skin by increasing blood flow and thus the level of nourishing nutrients it receives, to ensure that your complexion is truly glowing.

- **MATCHA** comprises 100 per cent natural green tea leaves, ground into a fine powder that's packed with lovely vitamins and minerals. In particular, it contains flavonoids, which protect skin from antioxidant damage and keep it looking youthful and clear!

- **MORINGA** brings an enormous number of benefits to the skin. It's sky-high in antioxidants, containing huge concentrations of vitamins and minerals.

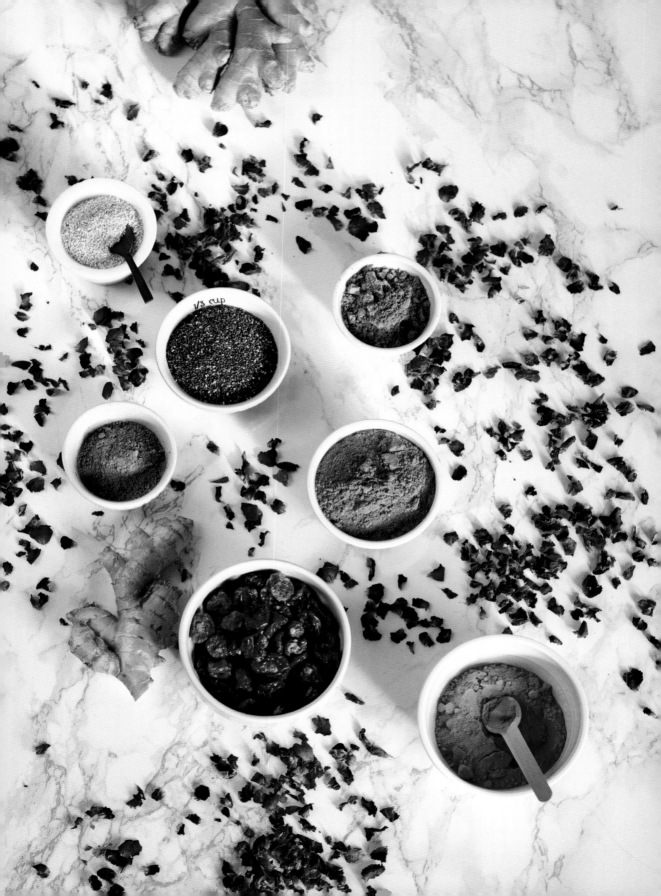

FOOD ENEMIES
of the SKIN

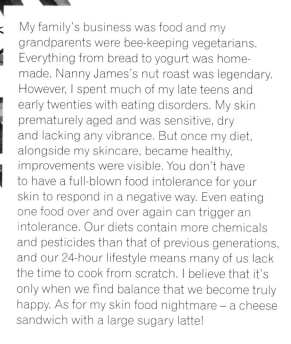

I spent much of my late teens and early twenties with eating disorders. My skin prematurely aged and was sensitive.

My family's business was food and my grandparents were bee-keeping vegetarians. Everything from bread to yogurt was home-made. Nanny James's nut roast was legendary. However, I spent much of my late teens and early twenties with eating disorders. My skin prematurely aged and was sensitive, dry and lacking any vibrance. But once my diet, alongside my skincare, became healthy, improvements were visible. You don't have to have a full-blown food intolerance for your skin to respond in a negative way. Even eating one food over and over again can trigger an intolerance. Our diets contain more chemicals and pesticides than that of previous generations, and our 24-hour lifestyle means many of us lack the time to cook from scratch. I believe that it's only when we find balance that we become truly happy. As for my skin food nightmare – a cheese sandwich with a large sugary latte!

What to cut down on...

• **REDUCE THE GLUTEN**

A protein that's found in foods containing wheat, barley and rye, it's used as a thickening agent in many everyday foods such as sauces – so start reading those labels! I am gluten intolerant and Nanny James was coeliac. Gluten has been linked to many health issues as well as skin breakouts, patchy areas that look like hives, itchy skin rashes, bloating and puffiness – so if you're concerned, I'd advise making an appointment with your GP. Start by steering clear of bread, pasta, biscuits, cake, crackers, couscous, rye bread and pizza.

• **DITCH THE DAIRY**

Humans are the only mammals that continue to consume milk past babyhood. While I don't want to discourage anyone from eating dairy in moderation, it's best avoided if you suffer from acne and dry skin conditions. So that means cutting out milk, cheese, yogurt and ice cream. There are so many tasty milk alternatives, from almond, cashew and hazelnut milk to hemp, oat, rice and coconut, that you won't feel deprived! There are several reasons why dairy and acne can't be friends. Cow's milk contains large enzymes that can be difficult to digest.

My skin food nightmare – a cheese sandwich with a large sugary latte!

Goat's milk is more in line with human milk, so is digested more easily. Modern-day dairy farming relies upon producing vast quantities of milk, and hormones are given to cows to do this. These are present in the milk we consume on our cereal and in cups of tea and coffee, and they affect our own hormonal balance. We've explored the acne/hormone connection in chapter four. Dairy also contains a number of protein molecules that may cause intolerances and fats that can produce substances called prostaglandins. These have an inflammatory effect and imbalance our reproductive hormones and blood-sugar levels. If you do want to drink proper milk, full-fat from organic, grass-fed cows is the best option.

Whenever you remove something from your diet, you need to replace it with something else. So if you're acne-prone and cut out dairy, or if you just want to reduce your intake consider other calcium-rich foods that you may find more delicious! So dine out on dark green leafy vegetables (such as kale, watercress, spinach, chard, rocket and cabbage). Fill your supermarket trolley with broccoli, soft-boned fish such as tinned salmon, pilchards and anchovies, as well as nuts and seeds (especially almonds, Brazil nuts, sesame and sunflower seeds). Fruit has a higher sugar content than vegetables, so enjoy it in moderation. It doesn't matter how many supplements you take, how effective your skin products are or how many facials you have, if you're reacting to a food internally, you need to address the root cause.

- ## THE TELL-TALE SIGNS OF AN INTOLERANCE

If you're not sure if you're reacting to gluten, dairy or something else, the easiest way to find out the cause of your intolerance is to follow an elimination diet. Remove one thing at a time over the course of a month, then eat it again in a fairly high concentration. If your symptoms return within 72 hours, it's likely you're intolerant. Equally, should your symptoms disappear over the four-week period, it's best to eliminate it from your diet.

- ## WINE O'CLOCK

We've all had a hangover and seen how grey and dehydrated our skin looks the next day. Alcohol is not only a sugar but it also interferes with our sleep and has a hugely dehydrating effect on our skin. So yes, enjoy a glass of wine, but adding to the liver's toxic load is clearly not conducive to achieving a lovely youthful complexion. I'm often asked if red wine is better for us than other forms of alcohol. The answer is yes, because it contains a higher level of antioxidants. However, it's also full of sulphate preservatives, which can cause internal inflammation. This is the reason why you may look flushed after a couple of glasses – and why it's a definite no-no for people who suffer from rosacea. Think about having four alcohol-free days a week. If you know it's a key skin irritant, consider removing it from your diet completely. If you suffer from eczema, psoriasis or rosacea, opt for cleaner alcohols such as gin, vodka and tequila and mix them with soda or cranberry juice with lemon and lime instead of sweet fizzy mixers.

- ## I CAN STILL HAVE MY COFFEE, RIGHT?

Like alcohol, caffeine is broken down by enzymes in the liver. We all have different amounts of these enzymes, so it's common to find that while some people can't tolerate caffeine, others thrive on it. Caffeine is a stimulant and can put added pressure on our adrenals, which are the glands that control our response to stress. An overloaded adrenal gland uses up vital nutrients including B vitamins, vitamin C and magnesium, which are skin-boosting nutrients, so your skin isn't getting enough of them to stay healthy and vibrant. My advice is to swap your cup of coffee for a matcha green tea or redbush tea – and yes, I know it doesn't taste the same! However, even though matcha and green tea contain caffeine, research shows that they have a calming effect on the body and don't burden our adrenal glands.

The bittersweet truth *about* sugar

With so much attention highlighting the dangers of sugar – not to mention the sugar tax – the detrimental effect it has on our health is no longer a secret. Eating sugar drives up our insulin levels, upsetting the internal balance of our hormones and contributing to conditions such as polycystic ovary syndrome (PCOS) and endometriosis in women. However, the negative impact it has on our complexion is still not quite so widely known.

• SUGAR AND AGEING

Sugar is addictive, so cutting down is incredibly hard to do. But if that chocolate brownie starts calling when you hit the mid-afternoon slump, give yourself some extra resistance power by thinking that sugar is the ultimate ager. A moment on the lips is not just a lifetime on the hips – but on the skin too. New research has helped us understand why sugar has such an ageing effect on the skin. Collagen and elastin proteins are highly susceptible to an internal chemical reaction within the body called glycation that takes place between proteins and sugars. When it occurs, the same glucose that provides energy for our cells reacts with proteins (such as collagen, our skin's building blocks), resulting in the formation of lines and wrinkles and making the skin adopt a sallow, slack appearance – rather than looking plump and vibrant as you'd like it to.

• SUGAR AND ACNE

Does sugar really cause acne? The short answer is yes. As we already know from chapter four, imbalanced hormones and inflammation are two key contributors to breakouts. Sugar disrupts our hormonal balance by stimulating the pancreas to release insulin, which has the job of taking sugar into our cells. This puts extra stress on the liver to process the extra blood sugar. As the liver is responsible for processing hormones, the link between sugar and acne becomes clear. Sugar also promotes inflammation. A study in *The American Journal of Clinical Nutrition* took 29 young, healthy people and gave them either one or two cans of sugary drinks per day for three weeks. These were people who wouldn't normally have these types of drinks. After three weeks, the results were telling:

- Consuming one can per day caused inflammation levels to increase by 87%
- Consuming two cans per day, inflammation levels were up by 105%

Candida is another way sugar can trigger skin breakouts. Candida is yeast that lives in the skin and the digestive tract, thriving on sugar. When candida grows, it causes gut problems and affects how the body absorbs nutrients. Getting rid of candida involves following a strict sugar-free diet for a number of months.

• THE ACID/ALKALINE BALANCING ACT

When we talk about our internal acid/alkaline balance, we're not referring to the environment of our stomachs, which need to be highly acidic in order to digest food, but to the pH balance of the body as a whole after digestion has occurred. Lemons and limes, for example, are acidic but once metabolised they have an alkalising effect on the body. This is also true for many foods you would not expect, such as pineapples, raspberries, tangerines, watermelons and onions. As early as 1933, Dr. William Howard Hay from New York published *A New Health Era* in which he maintained that all disease is caused by 'self-poisoning' due to acid accumulation in the body. Our blood needs to have a pH of 7.4 and even just a small shift can cause death. The body's natural instinct is to survive, so it does its best to balance its pH levels, taking minerals, calcium, sodium, potassium and magnesium from vital organs and bones to neutralise the acid. Our body is approximately 20 per cent acidic and 80 per cent alkaline and to maintain this balance we want our diet to be made up of a similar ratio. The benefit to our skin comes from the body having a less inflammatory internal environment, where essential minerals and internal organs work well.

1 Proteins, cereals, sugars, coffee, alcohol and red meat are all acid-forming, so try and minimise your intake. Swap some of your red meat dishes for those containing lentils and beans to ensure you're still getting proteins.

2 Dairy is also acid-forming, so swap milk and cheeses for milk alternatives, such as coconut, yogurt, and goat's cheese.

3 Drink lots of water throughout the day. Add some lemon, mint or cucumber to make it more interesting.

4 Pack in fruit, vegetables, nuts and seeds.

5 Take alkalising greens powders such as spirulina and chlorella.

6 If you're eating whey protein as part of your fitness programme, find a plant alternative. Whey plays havoc with the body and is acid-forming.

7 Swap your jacket potato for a jacket sweet potato.

Why chocolate is good for your skin

Chocoholics rejoice! It's a commonly asked question – will chocolate worsen spots? The good news is that there's no scientific evidence to suggest chocolate actually does cause spots. However, the real connection comes from the added sugar, dairy and palm oil inside mass-produced chocolate, all of which are not good for our skin, blood-sugar levels, hormonal balance and gut health. Cocoa in its purer form is great for the skin. High in flavonols (antioxidants that help prevent the skin from UV damage), it also promotes blood flow and contains vitamins, antioxidants and minerals, with their associated anti-inflammatory benefits. Even the aroma can release seratonin inside the brain, our happy hormone that reduces stress. So if, like me, you love chocolate – make it good-quality, dark chocolate every time.

"

After all the words of warning, I'm all for treating yourself – it's rather boring to be good all the time! Being too restrictive with yourself brings its own stresses and really, a happy you is a beautiful you.

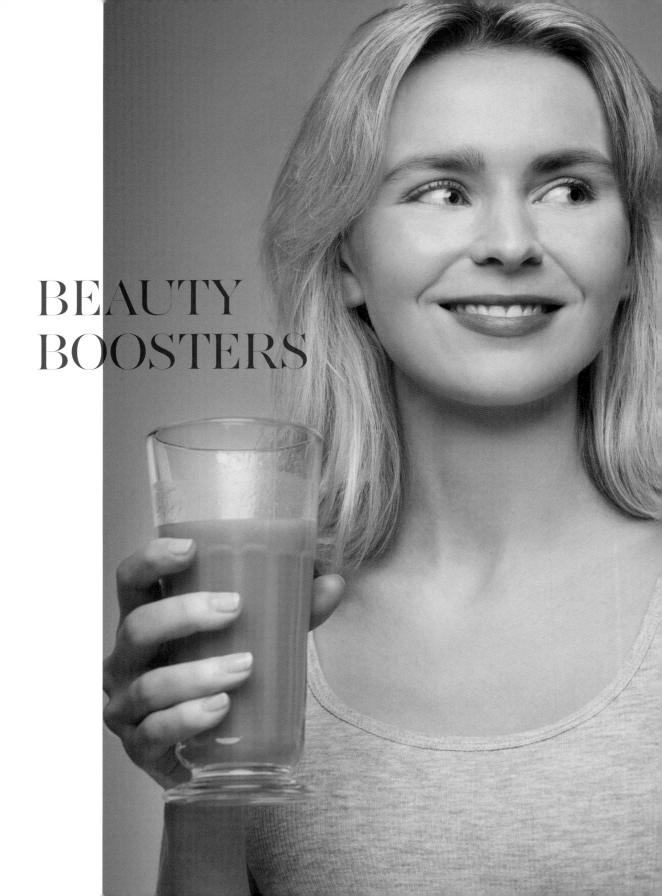

BEAUTY
BOOSTERS

On a daily basis our skin is subjected to damaging internal and external stressors. If we support our body with essential skin-loving nutrients every day we can give ourselves the best possible chance of keeping it healthy. I'm all about quick and easy when it comes to food, so I created these beauty boosters as an easy addition to your daily diets to give your skin the internal nutritional support and pick-me-up it needs.

These are all gluten- and dairy-free, plant-based foods to support your skin's health.

Beauty boosting juices

ANTI-AGEING SKIN TONIC WITH VITAMINS A AND C

1 orange
3 carrots
½ red pepper
small chunk of ginger
juice of ½ a lemon
½ teaspoon turmeric

optional boost:
baobab powder

Juice the orange, carrots, red pepper, ginger and lemon, then stir in the turmeric and booster separately.

SKIN SMOOTHING SMOOTHIE

¼ cucumber
200g pineapple, fresh or frozen
juice of ½ or whole lime, depending on taste
chunk of ginger
1 small avocado
a large handful of spinach or kale
boost: matcha, chlorella

Juice the cucumber, pineapple, lime and ginger. Smooth with all other ingredients in a blender.

CLEAN SKIN JUICE

½ cucumber
2 pears
¼ fennel or 2 sticks of celery
½ lemon
chunk of ginger
a large handful of spinach or watercress
a small handful of parsley

I juice all the ingredients; however, you can juice the cucumber, pear, fennel, lemon, ginger, then blend with the leaves.

Beauty boosting dips

HAPPY SKIN HUMMUS

Serves 4

1.x400g tin chickpeas
4 tablespoons tahini
1 garlic clove
3 tablespoons extra virgin olive oil
3½ tablespoons lemon juice
2 tablespoons water
a large handful of spinach
a small handful of coriander or basil
a small handful of parsley
salt and pepper

Blend all ingredients together until smooth or desired texture. Add more water if consistency is too thick.

AVOCADO, PEA AND MINT DIP WITH A KICK

Serves 4

1 ripe avocado
100g frozen peas, defrosted and drained
1 garlic clove
a small handful of mint
a small handful of watercress
juice of 1 lime
pinch of salt and pepper
2 tablespoons extra virgin olive oil
½ red chili, deseeded and finely chopped

Blend all ingredients together until smooth or desired texture. Add more water if consistency is too thick.

Beauty boosting balls

Makes 15–20

50g Brazil nuts
50g almonds
2 tablespoons pumpkin seeds
40g gluten-free oats or quinoa
8 dates
1 teaspoon cinnamon
2 tablespoons flaxseed, milled
pinch of Himalayan pink salt
4 tablespoons maple syrup or honey
4 tablespoons coconut oil, soft or liquid at room temperature
3 tablespoons raw cacao

In a blender grind the nuts and pumpkin seeds until fine. Add the oats or quinoa and blend again to refine the texture. Add the dates, cinnamon, raw cacao, flaxseed and salt and blend for a further 20 seconds. Place the mixture in a bowl, pour in the maple syrup or honey and the coconut oil.

Using your hands mix all the ingredients together for 3 to 5 minutes. Leave the mixture for 20 minutes so the oats and flax expand. Using your hands form the mixture into balls, pressing it tightly together. Store in an airtight container. They will last for up to two weeks.

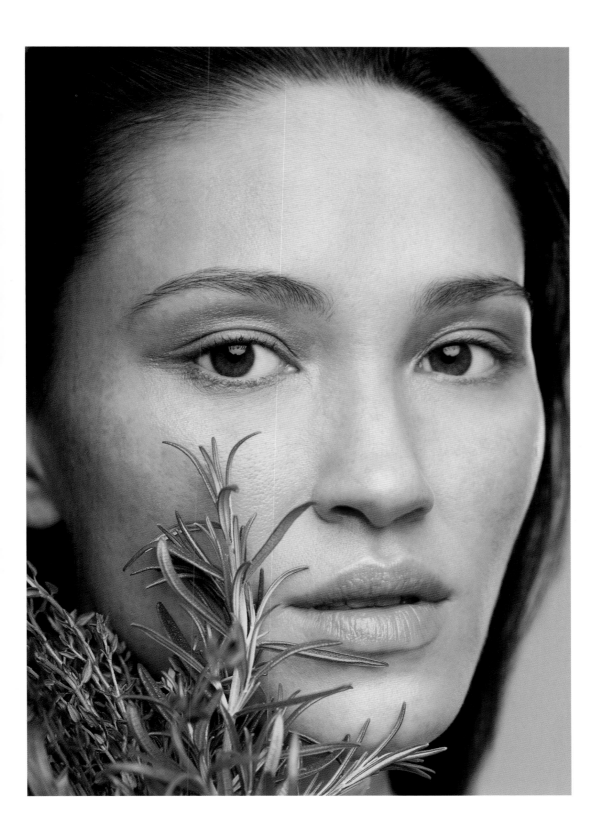

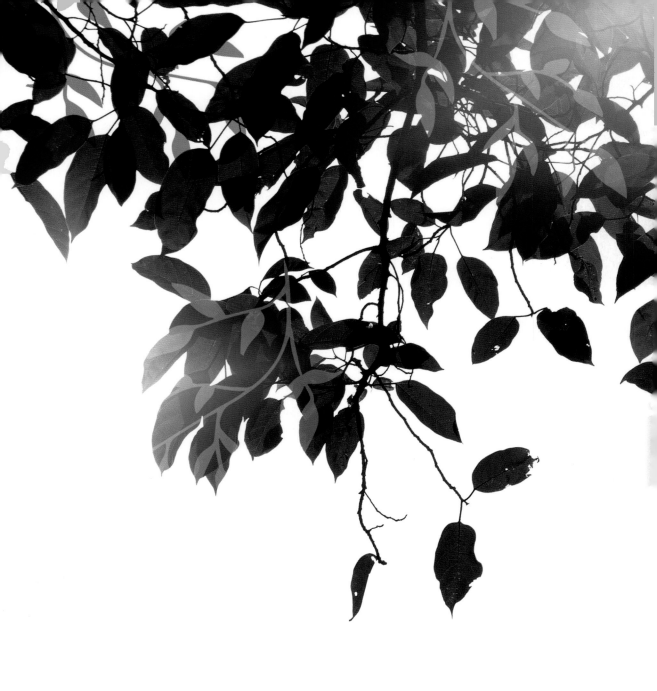

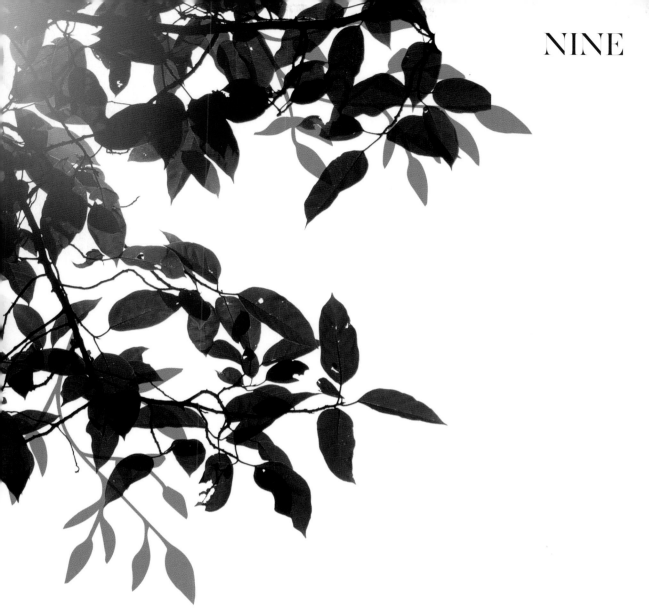

NINE

KITCHEN CUPBOARD REMEDIES

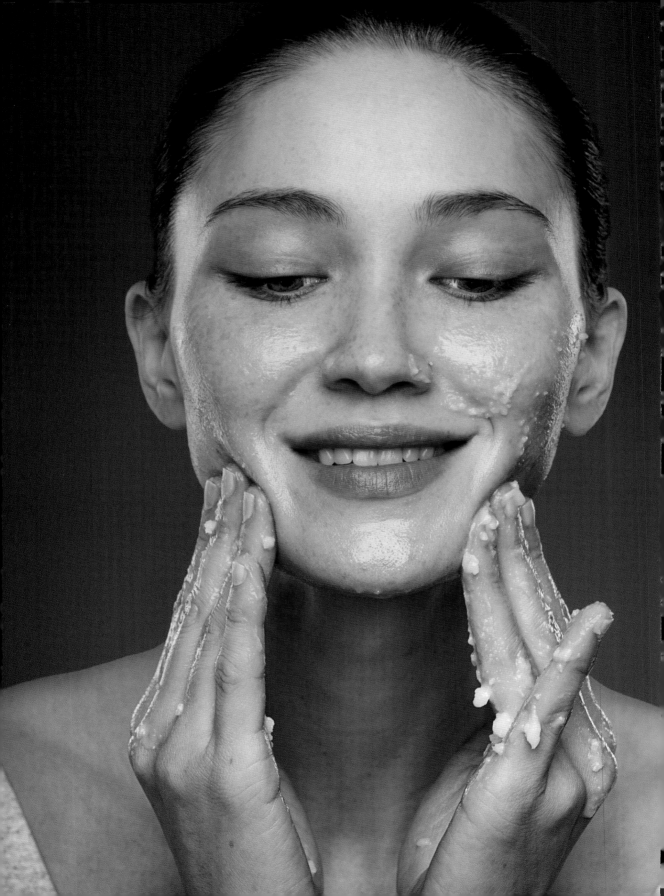

kitchen cupboard STOCK LIST

If it's good enough to eat, it's good enough to put on your skin. Our homes are full of skin-loving ingredients that are often used in the cosmetic industry and can easily be made into cost-effective skin treatments. Think about all the goodies inside your fridge, cupboards, medicine cabinet and garden – once you know which ones are good for you, you can tailor-make products that are best suited to your skin type.

From *the* cupboards

COCONUT OIL: an all-round skin star, it smells divine and its small molecular structure means it's easily absorbed. It's packed full of vitamin E, making it ideal for hydrating the skin, and also contains vitamin K, which is great for supporting and strengthening capillary walls, helping to reduce the appearance of dark circles and brightening the eyes. Its lauric acid content has antibacterial, anti-inflammatory benefits to soothe the soreness associated with eczema and psoriasis. It even melts away waterproof mascara. Try putting a small amount on a damp cotton-wool pad and wiping it over the whole eye area, including your brows.

APPLE CIDER VINEGAR: mostly acetic acid, it also contains lactic, citric and malic acid, vitamins, mineral salts and amino acids. With a pH similar to the skin, it helps restore your skin's natural acid/alkali balance and has a gentle exfoliating action. Drop some on to a cotton-wool pad and use it as a simple all-over skin-balancing toner.

HONEY: immensely healing, it has natural antibacterial and anti-fungal properties that have been shown to double in strength when diluted with water! Honey can heal burns and abrasions and because bacteria cannot live in it, honey is great for acne treatment and prevention. When it comes to anti-ageing, honey is full of antioxidants as well as being a fantastically soothing moisturiser. It helps to unclog pores and is the perfect addition to any home face mask.

SUSHI NORI: packed with vitamins and minerals, seaweed brings a whole host of skin benefits. Its anti-inflammatory properties make it great for spot-prone skin, while its vitamin C, selenium, iodine and vitamin B content increase cell metabolism, work to hydrate the skin and generally help slow down the ageing process. The vitamins in seaweed also ease the inflammation and redness associated with rosacea.

BLACK TEA: often underrated, it's packed full of the antioxidants vitamin B2, C and E and contains the minerals magnesium, potassium and zinc. The presence of tannins helps to protect the skin from environmental factors and boost cell regeneration.

GREEN & WHITE TEA: both are rich in vitamins and minerals, making them good all-rounders for problem and ageing skin. You can make skin-soothing ice cubes out of cooled tea. Glide one over the skin as and when you need to.

HERBAL TEAS: these are a really simple way of adding dried herbs into your recipes, particularly chamomile. Dampen and place a cool, wet teabag over the eyes to reduce puffiness, or add some to your bath for a soothing herbal infusion.

OLIVE OIL: full of both vitamins A and E and good for all skin types. If you're caught out at an impromptu sleepover without your cleanser, olive oil makes for a great alternative. Or you could simply add some olive oil to fine salt for a quick body scrub.

ALMOND OIL: a really lovely, gentle oil that's packed with vitamin E, yet is slightly lighter in texture than many other oils. This makes it great for rebalancing oily skin, while also being beneficial for sensitive and even babies' skin.

I love using almond oil on its own as a gentle eye-make-up remover on damp cotton-wool pads.

GROUND ALMONDS: bring all the benefits of the oil, plus it makes a great home exfoliant. Almond particles have a softness to them because of the natural oil content, so they hydrate the skin as they exfoliate dead cells away.

OATS: are incredibly versatile when it comes to caring for your skin. They're soothing, rich in minerals and make a lovely, gentle cleanser. They're often used in the treatment of eczema and to heal itchy, broken skin. When you add water to oats, they adopt a super-silky texture that feels great when applied to the skin.

SPIRULINA: is easily absorbed by the skin, supplying it with a potent source of protein (it has an incredible 60 to 70 per cent protein content). It aids in the removal of toxins just below the skin's surface and is one of the richest known sources of beta-carotene, a potent carotenoid. Carotenoids are the most powerful type of antioxidant with strong anti-ageing benefits. Also good for problem skin as it has a soothing, anti-inflammatory effect on the tissues and capillaries. It also absorbs water, making it ideal for skin-peeling and masks.

RICE FLOUR: a gentle ingredient with skin-lightening and antioxidant benefits, rice flour has a super-gentle but thorough exfoliating effect and has been used in Asia for centuries to treat inflamed skin. Its chemical structure is similar to that of the ceramides (a fat that helps hold moisture) in your skin.

BAKING SODA: not just for baking cakes, it's an alkaline substance that can help rebalance the skin's pH level and has antibacterial, anti-fungal, antiseptic and anti-inflammatory properties, making it good for the treatment of acne, spots and inflammation.

TURMERIC: I add this spice to as many foods and home-made face masks as possible. It's often used in Ayurvedic medicine for its antibacterial, anti-fungal and anti-inflammatory properties, which make it ideal for the treatment of acne and irritated skin. Just be careful as it can stain your skin. If you mix your turmeric mask with yogurt, there's much less chance of staining.

CINNAMON: not only does it smell amazing and evoke memories of Christmas, but it also contains calcium, fibre, iron and manganese. Cinnamon has astringent and antibacterial properties that soothe irritated skin. I like using this to give a glow and stimulate blood flow.

From *the* fridge

Natural yogurt: has a creamy texture and is super-cooling. It's a great ingredient to add to any home-made face mask to benefit all skin types. Yogurt contains lactic acid, which is an AHA that dissolves dead skin cells. This gentle exfoliation not only helps to create a natural glow and prevent breakouts, but works to diminish the appearance of lines and wrinkles.

Aloe vera: a skincare essential. Bringing cooling, soothing and hydrating benefits, it's no wonder that it's used in so many well-known commercially produced products. If you have an aloe plant, simply cut a piece off and apply it directly to wounds, minor burns and sensitive skin. Aloe vera juice fresh from the fridge can be applied to dry cotton-wool pads and wiped over sensitive areas. It also contains a whole host of antioxidants, making it an excellent anti-ageing ingredient.

From *the* medicine cabinet

- **WITCH HAZEL:** rich in tannins and has skin-balancing benefits with a mild astringent effect.
- **ESSENTIAL OILS:** some of my favourites include:
- **TEA TREE:** which has antibacterial, anti-fungal properties.
- **LAVENDER:** an antiseptic with healing powers.
- **CHAMOMILE:** both soothing and calming.

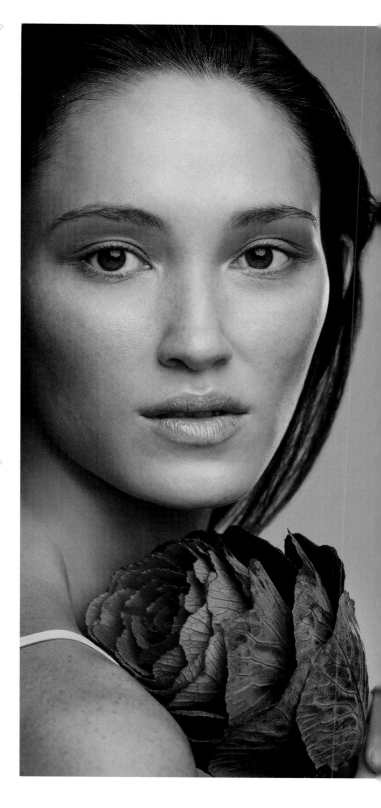

From *the* fruit bowl

CHERRIES: packed with antioxidants such as vitamin C and have skin-protecting properties.

PINEAPPLE: rich in vitamins, minerals and enzymes that have a gentle exfoliating and brightening action.

RASPBERRIES: are a relative of the rose. They're packed with vitamin E and other antioxidants, making them great for hydration and preventing the signs of ageing.

AVOCADO: mashed up, it can be simply used on its own for a soothing hydrating mask or added to most other ingredients. It's a great all-rounder for dry, delicate skins as it contains huge amounts of vitamin E, EFAs and nourishing, soothing oils.

BANANA SKIN: yes – the skin, not the flesh! The skin contains many beneficial nutrients for those suffering from acne, including essential antioxidants such as vitamins A, B, C and E, zinc, magnesium and iron, which all support and calm the skin when breakouts arise. Banana skin also works as a natural exfoliant, helping to keep pores clear, plus contains antibacterial enzymes that hydrate and heal. It also contains starch, which helps to absorb excess oil. Mashed banana flesh can also be used on the face, but due to its slippery texture, it can be difficult to apply and keep in place!

PAPAYA: contains an enzyme called papain, which naturally exfoliates the skin, while brightening, lightening, smoothing and repairing it. It's often used in professional clinics as a fruit enzyme peel ingredient. It contains lots of antioxidants and the pulp is fantastic for hydrating the surface of the skin.

CUCUMBER: is made up of 95 per cent water. Cooling, soothing and packed with hydrating liquid, it also contains essential vitamins such as K and C.

make at home

NATURAL WASHING GRAINS

Japanese washing grains (traditionally ground adzuki or mung beans) have been used for centuries and were made famous in the 1980s by Anita Roddick of The Body Shop. I've brought the recipe up to date with the addition of other beneficial ingredients – a blend of oats, nuts, seeds and herbs that have been ground down to a fine powder – to create a perfect, all-round exfoliating cleanse. They are suitable for all skin types, you can simply use 1 teaspoon in the palm of your hand and add water, or pop some of the powder into your daily cleanser for an extra skin-buffing boost.

2 tablespoons oats
2 tablespoons adzuki or mung beans
1 teaspoon milk powder
1 teabag black tea
1 tablespoon ground flaxseed
1 tablespoon ground almonds
2 tablespoons rice flour

Place all the ingredients in a coffee grinder or food processor and blend until all the ingredients become a soft, fine powder.

Decant the powder into a dry container with a lid, such as a jam jar. It will keep for six to 12 months if you keep it dry.

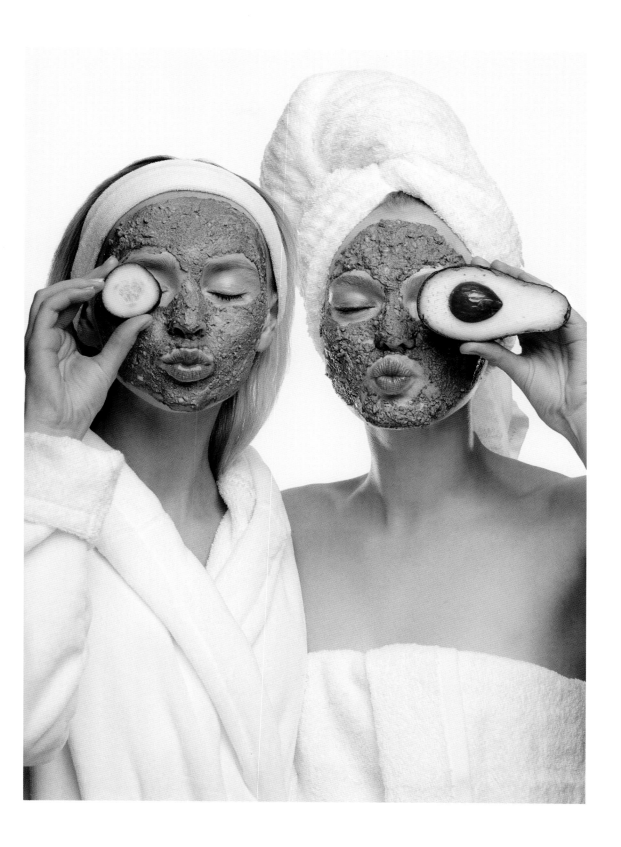

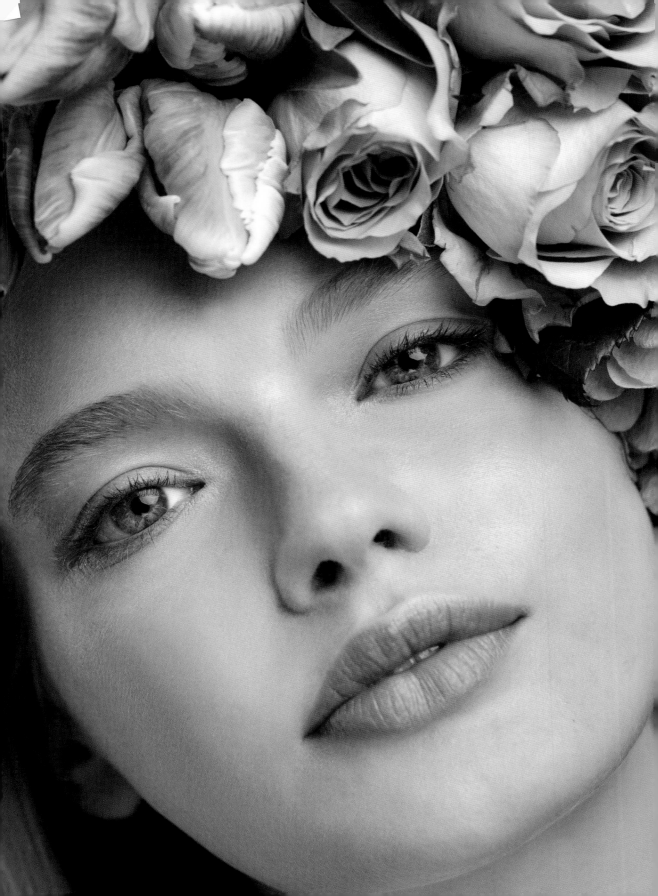

From *the* garden

Herbs and flowers have been used for centuries within the natural health and skincare industry. Here are just a few of my favourites. Add a handful to any of your home-made face masks to give your skin an extra boost.

- **DAISY:** really well-suited to blemished and oily skins and a great tissue repairer.

- **DANDELION:** a natural detoxifier, anti-inflammatory and soothing with mega amounts of antioxidants.

- **CHAMOMILE:** a skin soother with healing, anti-inflammatory properties.

- **LEMON BALM:** from the mint family, it's full of anti-inflammatory properties and is a rich source of tannins. It's brilliant for speeding up the skin's healing process and is often used as a herbal treatment of herpes, shingles and skin inflammation.

- **PANSIES:** pretty little flowers that are good for balancing the skin and aiding the detoxification process.

- **LAVENDER:** with soothing, antiseptic, calming and antibacterial properties, lavender is full of skin benefits. I love collecting lavender heads and drying them so I have a ready supply to use all year round.

- **MARIGOLD:** also known as calendula, these bright orange and yellow flowers are multifunctional when it comes to skin health and are used in numerous skincare products. They contain many antioxidants and have anti-inflammatory benefits. Add to juices when picked fresh. Marigold tea is also supposed to be good for menstrual cramps.

- **ROSE PETALS:** have a balancing effect on the skin. If you can get hold of damask rose, all the better.

- **ROSEMARY:** a mild astringent with blood-stimulating benefits.

- **SAGE:** soothing and a great skin supporter, bringing both nurturing and antibacterial benefits.

The best *at home* ingredients

These are all ingredients you're likely to have in your kitchen cupboards, but as well as tasting good, they all have proven benefits when applied topically to the skin.

1 KITCHEN CUPBOARD EXFOLIANTS FOR THE FACE

- Oats
- Rice flour
- Baking soda
- Citrus fruit
- Ground almonds
- Natural yogurt

2 SKIN MOISTURISERS

- Avocado oil
- Coconut oil
- Almond oil
- Olive oil
- Sesame oil

3 ANTI-INFLAMMATORY INGREDIENTS

- Turmeric
- Aloe vera
- Cucumber
- Natural yogurt
- Honey
- Spirulina

4 SKIN BALANCERS

- Honey
- Witch hazel
- Banana
- Rosemary
- Lavender
- Sushi sheets
- Natural yogurt
- Spirulina

5 SKIN BRIGHTENERS

- Cinnamon
- Lemon
- Apple cider vinegar
- Apples
- Strawberry
- Papaya
- Pineapple
- Cayenne pepper

6 SKIN LIGHTENERS

- Potato
- Lemon
- Lime

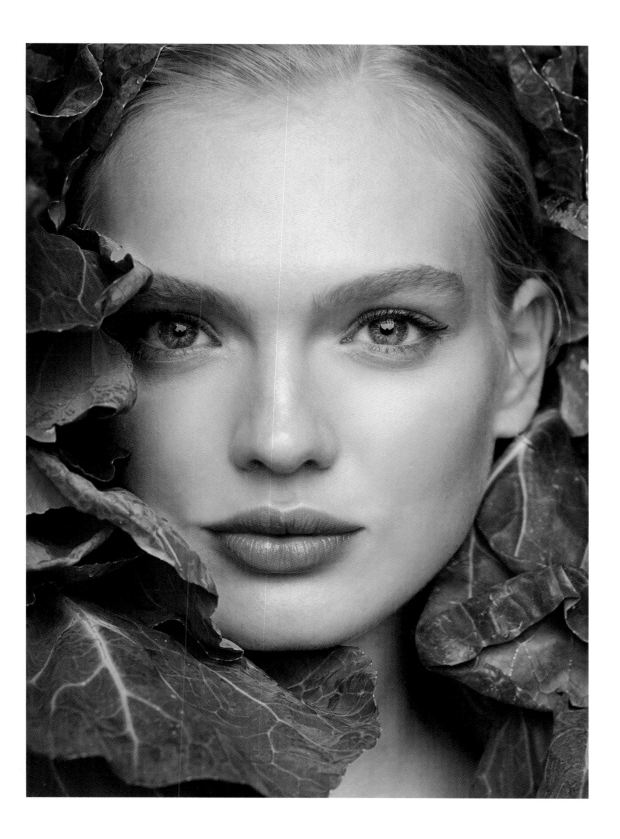

SKIN TONICS

Natural facial tonics are easy to make and can be tailored to suit your skin's needs. If kept in the fridge, they can last for up to two weeks, plus if applied cold, they have double the refreshing impact. Simply place the herbs, tea, plants or flowers in a teapot, pour over boiled filtered water, leave to infuse for a minimum of 30 minutes, then strain into a glass jug. Once cool, add 3 tablespoons witch hazel, which acts as a mild astringent and also helps to keep your tonic fresh for longer. Alternatively, adding 2 tablespoons aloe vera will provide some extra skin-soothing and hydrating benefits.

Skin Hydrating & Restoring Spritz

a couple of sprigs of fresh chamomile or half the contents of a chamomile teabag
a small handful of fresh rose petals or 1 tablespoon of dried rose petals
1 fresh head of lavender
1 white teabag

Perfect Balance Floral Skin Tonic

a few heads or small sprigs of:
    daisies
    lemon balm
    marigolds
    pansies
    rosemary

I suggest using a large teapot or small saucepan. You may wish to freeze some in ice-cube trays and defrost them as and when you need them over the course of the following month.

De-puffing Eye Compress

¼ cucumber
½ potato
2 tablespoons aloe vera
2 tablespoons witch hazel

Simply juice the cucumber and potato, then add the aloe vera and witch hazel. Keep it in a container with a lid in the fridge. When you're ready to use it, cut a cotton-wool pad into two half-moon shapes and soak them in the liquid before placing one under each eye. You can continue with your household tasks as they'll stick to your face! If you want to treat the whole eye area, soak two more cotton-wool pads, lie back, place them over the eyes and relax for 15 minutes.

Tired Eye Cure

If you don't have a juicer, simply blend all the above ingredients together until smooth, then add ½ teaspoon of matcha green tea and a small sprig of rosemary. Decant the liquid into an ice-cube tray and freeze. Wipe a cube over and around the whole eye area as needed.

Banana Peel Spot Treatment Face Mask

peel of 2 bananas
1 teaspoon natural yogurt
1 tablespoon apple cider vinegar
1 tablespoon honey

So as not to waste any of the flesh, simply freeze the skin of a banana whenever you eat one. I've combined it with skin-healing honey to reduce inflammation and bring natural antibacterial effects. The apple cider vinegar balances the complexion's pH, while the natural yogurt calms, soothes and gently exfoliates. Ideally, use overripe bananas. Blend all the ingredients together and apply the mixture to your face. Use daily to get the benefits and keep in the fridge. Although the mask will go dark it can still be used for 3 days after. As you wash it off after 20 to 30 minutes, you may feel a slight tingling sensation, which is normal.

Brightening Papaya Pineapple Face Peel

½ pineapple, skin removed and sliced
a large chunk of papaya, skin and seeds
¼ sweet potato or 2.5cm slice of pumpkin

Blend all the ingredients together. This mask has a real 'wow' effect, so is the perfect way to brighten the skin before a big night out. The blend of enzymes and natural AHAs really exfoliates, smooths and brings a new-found radiance to the skin. It feels like a mild skin peel and may cause a slight itching and tingling effect. It will set on the skin, so just splash on a small amount of water and then rinse it off with a cloth. You can repeat this once a week. If you have time, multi-mask and follow it with a lovely, soothing mask recipe.

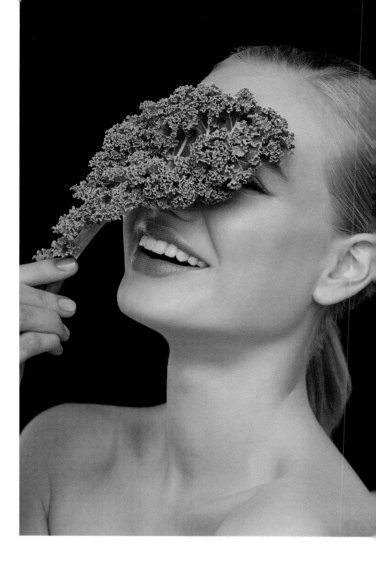

Skin Restoring Face Mask

½ teaspoon turmeric
2 tablespoons natural yogurt
1 tablespoon almond oil
3 lemon leaves
1 teaspoon aloe vera
1 tablespoon oats

Blend all the ingredients together. This will produce a thick yellow mask that can be applied to the face with a cotton-wool pad and left on for ten minutes.

Chocolate Orange Avocado Nourishing Mask

1 heaped teaspoon raw cacao powder
1 avocado
1 tablespoon honey
¼ orange, including skin
1 tablespoon aloe vera, optional

Place all the ingredients in a blender and mix until really smooth. This mask can be used as a neck and décolletage mask. It can be kept in the fridge for a few days and will make enough to share with friends. The orange has a brightening effect, while the cacao restores the skin, the avocado nourishes and the honey heals. Leave it on for up to 30 minutes. It will set slightly and need softening with water before you remove it with a cloth.

Super Greens Balancing Mask

1 teaspoon spirulina
1 tablespoon honey
2 tablespoons natural yogurt
1 teaspoon apple cider vinegar

Mix all the ingredients together. Both the apple cider vinegar and spirulina rebalance the skin.

Soothing Antioxidant Rose Petal Mask

1 large handful fresh, or 2 heaped
    tablespoons, of dried rose petals
½ teaspoon coconut oil
2 tablespoons natural yogurt
6 cherries, stones removed, or raspberries
1 white or green teabag, soaked
2 tablespoons honey

Mix all the ingredients in a blender, apply to the face and leave on for 20 minutes.

Skin Balancing Seaweed Face Mask

2 sheets sushi nori
apple cider vinegar (if you have problem skin)
    or rose or orange blossom water (if you
    have sensitive skin)
green or white tea

If you're not a fan of the smell of the seaside, then this might not be one for you. However, it is a great mask for sensitive and unbalanced skins. Make a mug of tea and leave it to cool until it's lukewarm. Pour this into a deep plate or large bowl. Add the apple cider vinegar or floral waters and soak the nori sheets for 1 minute. Carefully rip them into large pieces and place over your face. Leave them on for 20 minutes. As an alternative, soak 2 sheets and place them in a blender with natural yogurt and honey. This will make a cool, creamy, easy-to-apply face mask that rebalances the skin.

Spicy Skin Brightening Mask for Problem Skin

½ teaspoon turmeric
½ teaspoon spirulina
½ teaspoon cinnamon
½ teaspoon bicarbonate of soda

Blend all the powders together and store in an airtight pot. When you're ready to use it, mix the powder blend with your choice of natural yogurt (for a freshening, brightening effect) or mashed avocado (for nourished, hydrated skin). Leave it to dry and feel it tighten on the skin. Add some water and use it as a scrub, as the coarse spice particles remain on the skin and act as a smoothing scrub.

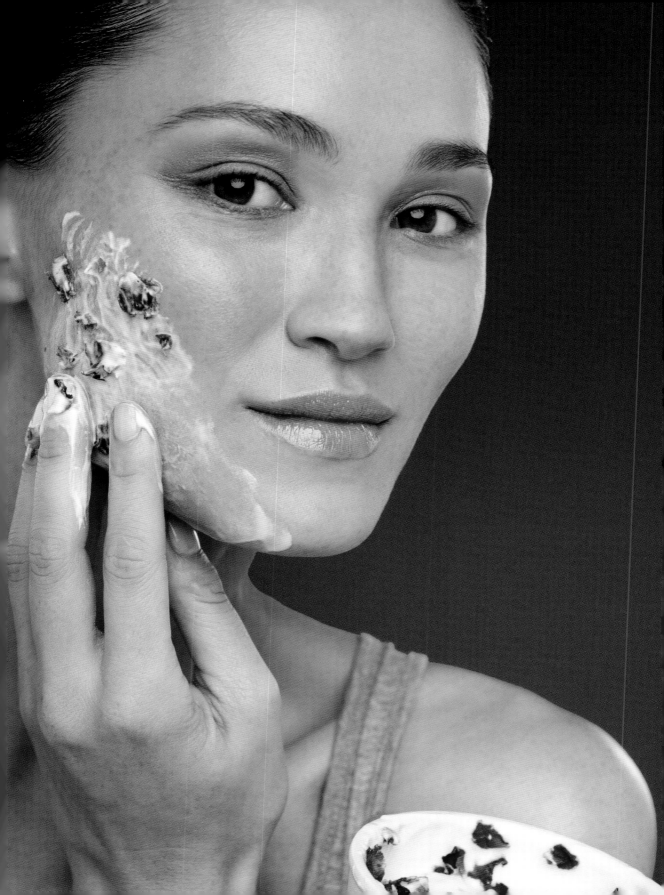

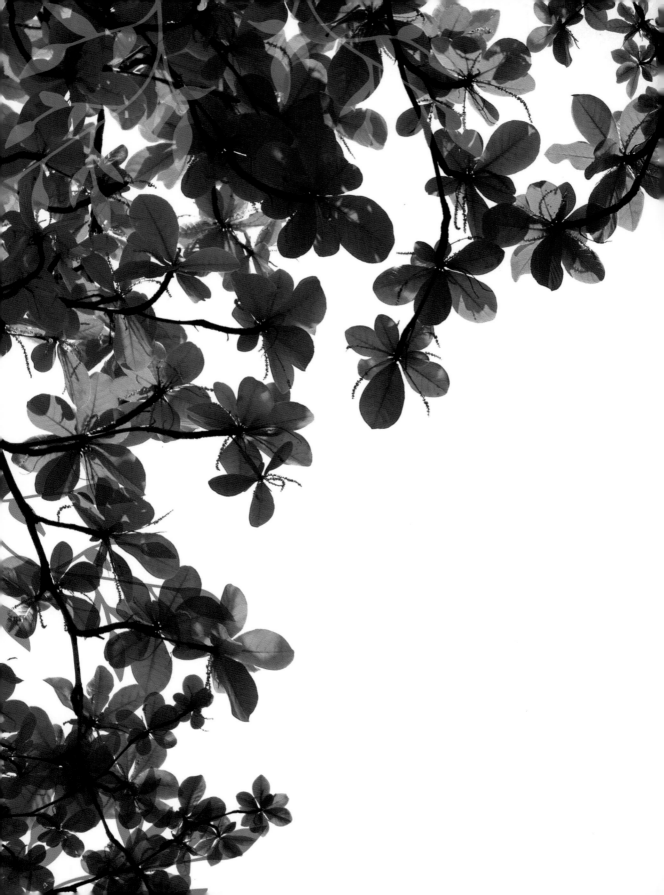

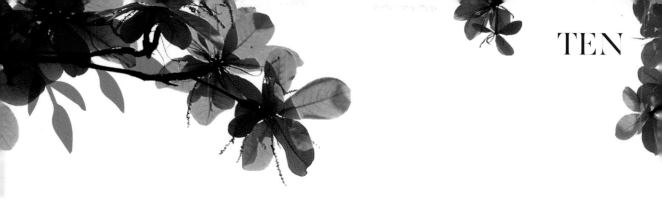

a ROAD MAP *to* FACIALS

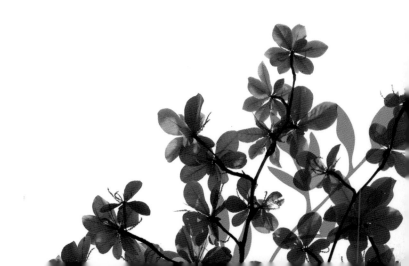

Being epileptic I'm unable to have any electric or light machines and I feel too uncomfortable to use Botox or fillers. I'm so pleased to have met Abigail. She has magic hands – just one treatment of her face massage makes an incredible difference, it's so relaxing and my cheekbones and eyebrows feel lifted and tighter and my wrinkles are smoothed – so much so I had a close relative ask if I'd had Botox. They didn't believe me when I said 'no'

KAREN J GERRARD – CLIENT

In the early years of my career my passion was for a hands-on, holistic approach to skincare. My work as a sports massage and holistic therapist in an Ayurvedic spa in the Cotswolds had a huge influence on my methods. I learnt Chinese, Japanese, Indian and Western facial and body therapies. As my knowledge grew and my skin began to age, I started to research technology that could work alongside my techniques. My philosophy is combining great skincare, nutrition and lifestyle practices, which you will find throughout this book, with effective new treatments and technology. One facial can bring about visible improvements but regular treatments can be the difference between good skin and great skin – with long-lasting results. Even if you don't suffer from a chronic skin condition, your complexion will benefit hugely from the attention of an expert facialist. The results and comfort factor will depend upon the practitioner, so choose carefully.

The life cycle of a facial

- IMMEDIATELY: after 48 hours, skin looks visibly hydrated, radiant and glowing.

- THREE TO SIX DAYS LATER: circulation has been boosted, skin looks and feels healthy. Some pimples may be brought to the surface. Ideally, exfoliate thoroughly one week after treatment.

- ONE TO TWO WEEKS LATER: cell turnover has been boosted and skin still feels healthy.

- FOUR TO SIX WEEKS LATER: time for your next treatment. New cells that benefited from your last facial have now gone through a whole turnover cycle.

Massage

All good facials should incorporate some element of facial massage. The exceptions are specific treatments such as peels or LED. Massage works on both a physical and an emotional level and has the ability to naturally lift, sculpt and drain the face of puffy fluid using my techniques.

Clients who, for medical reasons, I'm unable to treat with machinery particularly love the results of my lifting massage methods.

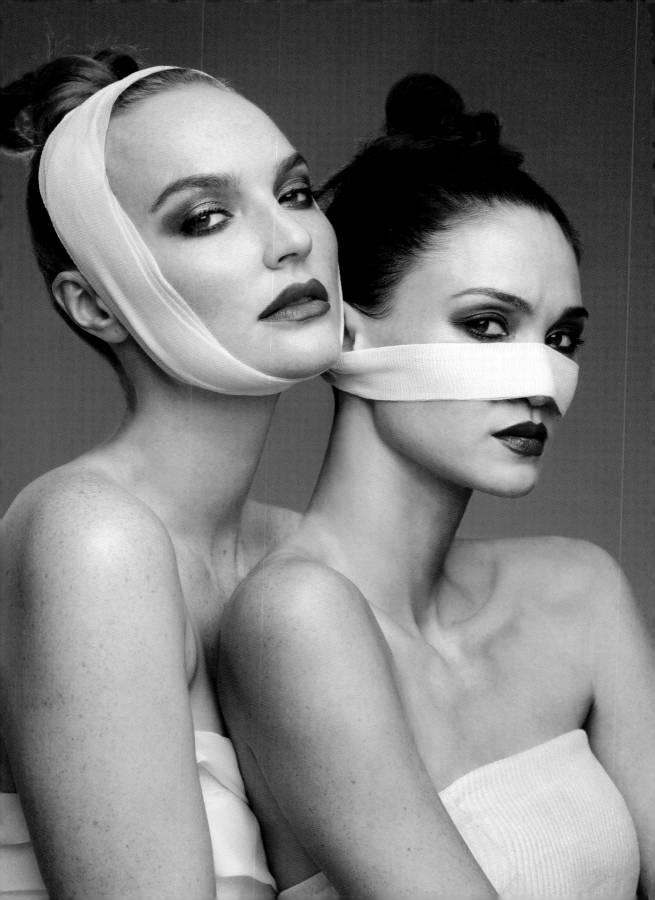

Are peels right for you?

The word 'peel' can evoking memories of Samantha's disastrous one in *Sex and the City*. But that red rash of a reaction was down to old-school methods. Skin peels have come on leaps and bounds since then and can be game changers.

- ### WHAT THEY DO

Their aim is to exfoliate (remove) cells from the surface and correct imperfections. They also speed up collagen production to give you vibrant, smooth skin. Peels generally work within the epidermis (the outer layer of the skin). The kind of stronger peels, such as a Jessner Peel, often used for severe acne and deep ageing lines, work within the dermis to force the skin into creating a whole new layer. They can result in redness, swelling and full-skin shedding, so require downtime of one to two weeks. They are not my chosen method of treating the skin. Those with thin, delicate, reactive skins would do best to steer clear of them.

- ### THE DIFFERENT TYPES

The two key points of difference are:
1. How deep the peel will penetrate.

2. What the intended action is.

These points are determined by the type of acid, its concentration, the pH of the peel, how many layers are applied to the skin and the length of time it's left on for. In general, the deeper the peel, the more downtime, disruption to the skin and risk of prolonged healing.

- ### PH LEVELS

It's possible to have a 40 per cent peel that has a low pH, which means its impact will be minimal, and a 20 per cent peel that has a high pH, which means it can be more aggressive. The pH scale runs from 1 (acid) to 14 (alkaline). The pH of skin is 5.5, which is slightly acidic, and is why soap, with its pH of 8–9 has a drying effect. Water has a pH of around 7; face wipes have one of around 10, and alcohol has a pH of around 3 to 4. The lower the pH, the deeper the peel will penetrate.

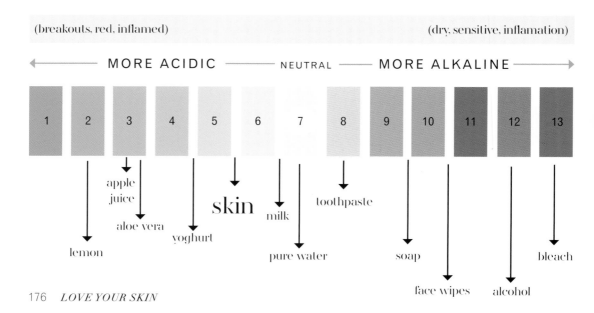

(breakouts, red, inflamed)   (dry, sensitive, inflamation)

← MORE ACIDIC —— NEUTRAL —— MORE ALKALINE →

| 1 | 2 | 3 | 4 | 5 | 6 | 7 | 8 | 9 | 10 | 11 | 12 | 13 |

lemon · apple juice · aloe vera · yoghurt · skin · milk · pure water · toothpaste · soap · face wipes · alcohol · bleach

- ## ENZYME PEELS – THE PERFECT PRE-EVENT BOOST

These are from a plant source and are part of the peeling family (see chapter six). They are the gentlest type of peel and create very little sensation on the skin, so they're usually suitable for all skin types, including sensitive ones. Perfect for a quick brightening, skin smoothing and freshening-up, they're great for all-round skin health. They work in a Pac-Man type of way, gently eating up and dissolving dead cells on the surface of the skin. After an enzyme peel I find skin looks and feels radiant for a number of days.

- ## ALPHA-HYDROXY ACIDS (AHAs)

These are naturally occurring acids that help to exfoliate the surface, as well as speed up skin cell turnover. They have a deeper and longer-lasting impact than enzymes. Many brands have professional peels that are made up of a combination of AHAs to give a rounded result. They can often be found in your home skin products, over-the-counter exfoliants, cleansers and masks in lower concentrations (see chapter 6).

- ## GETTING THE BEST FROM YOUR PROFESSIONAL PEEL

Some peels are perfectly safe and effective to have with no previous skin preparation. They're often included as part of general facials as an effective method of exfoliating and boosting the skin. They're great if you need a quick freshen-up before attending a special event. I would recommend using a gentle cleanser and no exfoliant at home for at least two days after the treatment and it's essential you wear an SPF. Other peels may require you to have prepped the skin with certain products, so that you get the best result and minimal downtime. Cut out any retinol products one week before the treatment and only resume using them at least seven days afterwards or you're likely to experience sensitivity.

After your peel, avoid perfumed skincare and high levels of aromatherapy as these may irritate the skin. Cut out strong cleansing washes that contain AHAs, as well as antibacterial ingredients such as salicylic acid. Instead, opt for gentle, soothing cleansers for three to four days. You might need to factor in your work-life schedule for medium-strength peels – your skin might be slightly flushed immediately after, then look vibrant for a few days. By day four to five, it might feel a little dry and itchy but by day seven to ten, it will be more vibrant than ever. If you're having a course of peels these are usually staggered two weeks apart to maximise results.

Skincare peeling ingredients

- LACTIC ACID: SOUR MILK: good for hydration

- GLYCOLIC ACID: SUGAR: good exfoliator

- MANDELIC ACID: bitter almonds – oily – problem, antibacterial larger molecule than lactic

- CITRIC ACID: LEMONS: good for pigmentation

- AZELAIC ACID: apples – good for breakouts

- KOJIC ACID: mushrooms – good for pigmentation

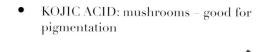

Radiofrequency (RF):
the contour refiner

RF is great for boosting collagen, increasing skin firmness and redefining the facial contours. It was originally part of the more medical side to beauty and could cause dermal burns, but has developed into a safe, effective method with no recovery time. It stimulates the body's natural healing response by heating the skin to approximately 40°C to increase collagen production, without harming the surrounding tissue. It tightens collagen fibres and gives instantly visible results. I love this as a pre-event treatment. It continues to increase collagen production over the following four to six weeks, so it really is a facial that continues to work while you sleep! There are different types of machines with a different number of electrodes in the head. I prefer the multipolar type, which is highly effective and doesn't cause discomfort. My clients adore this method – they say it feels like a hot-stone face massage but with incredible lifting results.

THE BENEFITS
- Tightens skin
- Softens fine lines
- Firms facial contours, neck, jaw and cheekbones
- Brightens and improves the overall appearance and radiance of the skin

Microcurrent:
the face's personal trainer

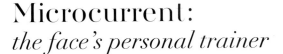

This technique improves muscle firmness, lifts, re-defines facial contours and boosts collagen production. The technology was originally used within the medical field for the treatment of Bell's palsy and strokes to stimulate and re-educate the facial muscles, but is now used for its beauty benefits and skin healing too. I particularly like microcurrent treatments as they're suitable for all skin types. They use a low-level electrical current to stimulate the body's natural ability to improve cell energy. However, the current doesn't interfere with our own electrical fields, making it totally safe. Some machines give no sensation while others give a mild tingling feeling. This treatment has no downtime – but yields big results! An ideal course is performed once a week for eight treatments. It's also a great addition to your monthly facial treatment. Different machines use different patterns of microcurrent with varying penetration abilities and effects.

THE PHYSICAL EFFECTS:
- Increases cell energyadenosine triphosphate (ATP) by 500 per cent.
- Increases fibroblast activity, boosting collagen production by up to 60 per cent.
- Increases protein synthesis by approximately 30 per cent.
- Increases cell absorption by approximately 40 per cent.

THE BENEFITS
- Lifts and tones the muscles
- Increases cell energy
- Is suitable for even sensitive skin

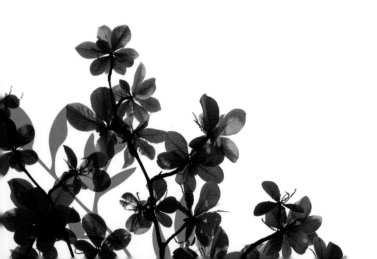

Microdermabrasion:
the skin smoother

This has a smoothing effect on the surface of the skin, improves product absorption and reduces the appearance of fine lines. The machine exfoliates and smooths by working on the uppermost layers of skin. It also stimulates a healing response and accelerates new cell growth. This means that it helps any products you apply afterwards to penetrate more easily and efficiently.

THE DIFFERENT TYPES:
1. Using a diamond tip involves rubbing a fine exfoliating head with a fine sandpaper type tip over the surface of the skin to exfoliate the surface.

2. Crystal microdermabrasion involves blasting tiny particles of aluminium oxide, sodium bicarbonate or salt across the surface of the skin using a small hand-held probe. This probe has a vacuum-like suction effect to draw these particles back up and away from the skin and helps boost the action of the lymphatic system.

Vacuum suction:
the detoxer

This treatment supports drainage, reduces puffiness and assists in the removal of toxins and has been used for decades. A small amount of oil is applied before small glass heads are glided over the surface, causing a lifting and sucking effect. The extra support for the lymphatic system stimulates the delivery of fresh nutrients to the skin, making your complexion look brighter and more vibrant. This is generally a great treatment for all skin types – especially if you're in need of detox.

Oxygen:
the skin pick-me-up

This makes for plump, dewy skin. A good oxygen machine will infuse medical-grade oxygen into the skin via a head that pushes out a stream of pressurised oxygen. Every cell in our body requires oxygen to function, so this treatment acts as an immediate pick-me-up for the skin. I think of it as the perfect city skin treatment.

The oxygen also helps serums containing active ingredients to penetrate deeper into the skin, making them more effective. In Australia, this treatment has even been used to deliver chemotherapy to skin cancer patients. There's no downtime, it's safe, feels cooling and gives immediate results. Please be aware that some machines may have the word 'oxygen' in their name but only blow a low-level oxygen percentage, not that dissimilar to air, over the skin.

LED light therapy:
the skin healer

This boosts collagen production, skin healing, rejuvenation and has antibacterial benefits. It is a totally safe, non-invasive light treatment with no downtime. It works on the basis of the skin's ability to absorb light and triggers a natural response. The difference between treatments is the specific colours and wavelengths of light involved. Most widely used are red and blue light. When red LED light is absorbed, it has a regenerating effect, increasing cell energy, collagen and elastin for smoother, firmer skin. Blue LED light is effective for the treatment of acne, with antibacterial benefits and a reduction of sebum production. Different LED machines use different strengths, colours and wavelengths.

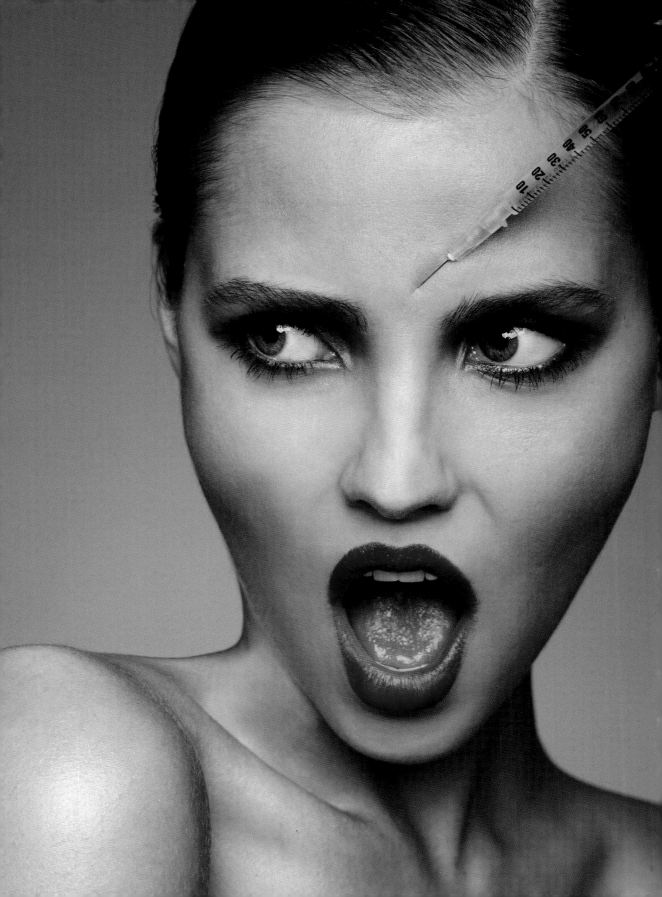

High frequency:
the acne reliever

This involves using a low-level electric current and a glass head filled with gas that emits a violet glow. It is swept over the skin's surface, causing little or no sensation, while bringing about an antibacterial effect. It helps increase blood flow and oxygenate the skin.

Galvanic:
the deep cleanser

During this treatment, a metal roller is used to apply a low-level electric current to the skin to help products penetrate deeper and soften the clogged material inside blackheads.

Skin needling:
the repairer

Also known as Collagen Induction Therapy, Dermaroller and micro-needling, it's based on the skin's natural ability to repair itself whenever it encounters physical damage. Immediately after the skin is injured, the body removes the damaged collagen, elastin and other structures and replaces them with freshly made, smooth components. It works by creating a 'controlled injury' to the skin surface, triggering its self-repair mechanisms. The micro-needles make invisible micro-channels in the skin, allowing serums, oils and other products to penetrate deeper. The use of longer needles may require a numbing cream, whereas shorter 0.3mm ones rarely need this. Over a period of months your skin becomes smoother, firmer and younger-looking. This is not a pampering facial and is not for everyone. The skin may feel warm, red and tight for four to eight hours afterwards, but any redness should go by the following day. No make-up for at least four hours post-treatment and please don't be tempted to purchase your own facial rollers from the internet – these need to be in the safe hands of a professional.

Fractional radiofrequency:
the skin smoother

This is a huge step up from skin needling – it adds the power of radiofrequency, which results in a deeper, more controlled method of stimulating collagen production, working to smooth and refine the surface and scarring. The machine head has around 100 tiny needles, which penetrate the skin and act as a path for the radio frequency to generate controlled heat within the dermis. A numbing cream may be required and some downtime, but the results are well worth it. When included in a combined treatment plan it is the ultimate in facial rejuvenation.

Botox:
the muscle blocker

Botox is a trademark for the botulinum toxin. It works by blocking the chemicals that cause our muscles to contract. Over many years, this repeated contraction leads to our beautiful character lines. Although still controversial, when performed properly, there's no risk of your face looking 'frozen' and it dramatically reduces the appearance of lines. The effects usually last for around three to four months. I wouldn't recommend it if you're pregnant, and if you are having Botox, looking after your skin through facials, massage and products is vital to keep the tissue healthy. At the end of the day, I just don't believe that a lack of muscle movement can be considered 'healthy'.

Fillers: *a risky option?*

Although increasingly popular, I've seen too many mistakes made with fillers. Clients often come to me after having had a bad experience that's left them with an undesirable result. I also believe that having too many fillers means that we're vulnerable to losing sight of what our true, individual beauty is – no matter how old we are.

Your QUESTIONS ANSWERED

There are some questions that crop up time and time again, but as more and more products, ingredients and technologies emerge, the answers can change. In this chapter I've answered some of the most common ones, but for up-to-date information you can also visit my website *abigailjames.com*.

Q. WHY DO I HAVE DARK CIRCLES UNDER MY EYES?

A. Dark circles are caused by a number of factors:

- Genes
- Dehydration
- Anaemia
- Tiredness
- Sluggish detoxification of waste and kidneys not eliminating effectively
- Too much sugar and starch in the diet
- A lack of exercise
- An indicator of low magnesium
- Nasal congestion and/or a sluggish lymphatic system (linked to certain medical conditions)
- Ageing as the skin becomes much thinner around the eyes
- Some medication

Q. HOW DO I TREAT MY DARK CIRCLES?

A. The dark colour comes from blood vessels close to the surface of the skin that dilate with certain conditions. If your circles aren't hereditary and you're getting enough sleep, then the best way to combat them is to support your body's digestion and detoxification processes (see chapter eight on liver support). Vitamin K is an essential nutrient for supporting the body's blood-clotting factors. Many eye creams contain vitamin K to strengthen capillary walls and prevent dark circles. Lymphatic drainage can also help as it removes waste and toxins. Magnetic therapy, often used by physiotherapists, has an ability to support tissue growth and speed healing, and has been shown to be beneficial in the reduction of dark circles.

Q. WHY ARE MY EYES SO PUFFY?

A. If it's not an allergic reaction to something, it could be connected to:

- A sluggish lymphatic system
- Hormonal changes
- Hereditary issues
- Poor diet
- Lack of exercise
- The wrong skincare
- Applying eye creams at night time
- Sinus congestion (which can be triggered by high levels of dairy)

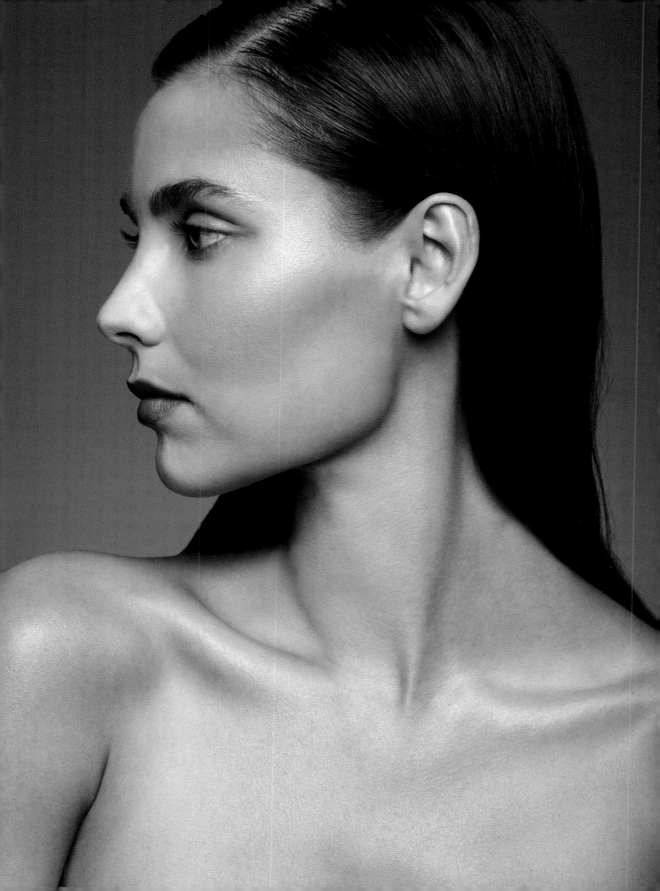

Q. WHAT'S THE BEST WAY TO TREAT MY PUFFY EYES?

A. Cutting out dietary toxins such as coffee and alcohol and drinking more water will go a long way. Try to go for a week without using any products around your eyes to ensure that it's not a reaction to a particular ingredient. When you've done that, apply your eye products in the morning, rather than at night. The skin around the eyes is ten times thinner than that of the rest of the face, so eye creams can sit in this delicate area and leave you with puffy eyes in the morning. It's a cliché but cold slices of cucumber or potato or damp nettle teabags really do work. Something with a slight astringent such as witch hazel is great for a quick freshen-up, so drop a little on a damp cotton-wool pad and wipe it over the eye area. You could also try massaging the area with the backs of cold spoons from the fridge. The cooling and draining effect will help disperse any fluid. Finally, cut your salt intake as this encourages water retention.

Q. WHY ARE MY PORES SO LARGE?

A. Pore size is hereditary. Drier skins tend to have finer pores, while oilier skins generally have larger ones. Our pores also get bigger as we age and unfortunately, there's no magic potion or treatment to drastically reduce their size. Keeping them clean with a good facial wash and regular exfoliation will help reduce build-up of sebum and blackheads, making them appear smaller. Professional treatments, including peels, micro-needling and fractional radiofrequency, will also help to reduce the appearance of large pores.

Q. WHAT CAN I DO ABOUT MY BLACKHEADS?

A. Ensure that you take your make-up off at the end of each day and avoid using face wipes as these often leave a residue. So too will a facial balm that contains mineral oils. Wash morning and night and include some AHA exfoliation and even a BHA exfoliation once a week. BHAs have the ability to clean out each pore and have both anti-inflammatory and antibacterial properties.

Try applying a clay mask once a week to help draw out impurities. But remember to add in some hydration so as not to over-strip the skin. You could also book in for a facial with steam and extraction.

Q. SHOULD I SQUEEZE MY BLACKHEADS AT HOME?

A. If you want to, but do it correctly, or you risk scarring your skin. I would always extract spots in the evening, as this allows around eight hours for any swelling and redness to calm down. Steam your skin first by filling a bowl with hot water, leaning your face over and covering your head with a towel for five minutes to ensure that your pores are soft, or extract spots after a hot shower. Pat your skin dry and wrap tissue around your index fingers. Without using your nails to dig into the skin, gently squeeze the pore from the sides, pushing underneath it as you do. Don't force it. If it doesn't go, then leave it and cool with something cold such as an ice cube.

Q. I HAVE SOME SCARRING ON MY FACE. CAN I GET RID OF THIS?

A. Eradicating scars is tricky. However, there are some methods that can reduce their appearance. Micro-needling, fractional radiofrequency and laser resurfacing all stimulate collagen production and 'fill in' the irregular texture around the scar. A course of such treatments is necessary and while they're not always comfortable, the results can be life-changing.

Q. I HAVE A BIG EVENT COMING UP AND A HUGE SPOT. CAN YOU HELP?

A. Apply an ice cube to the spot throughout the day to help reduce inflammation. Salicylic acid, zinc, tea tree, lavender and TCP all have antibacterial properties to help reduce the size and redness of the spot when applied directly to it. Unless it's a whitehead, don't squeeze it or you'll only make it worse. If you can see a whitehead, sterilise a needle or pin by holding it in a burning flame. Let it cool, then very carefully make a tiny pinprick on the white area. Wrap tissue around your fingertips and gently apply pressure either side of the spot. Don't force it – the pinprick has already given an exit point for the top part of white sebum. Apply your antibacterial product immediately afterwards and leave it alone. Don't be tempted to squeeze deeply or you'll make a mess!

Q. I'VE HAD A BAD REACTION TO A PRODUCT. WHAT SHOULD I DO?

A. Stop using all products as once you've had a reaction, your skin will be hypersensitive to anything you apply at this time. Use a floral water on a cotton-wool pad to gently cleanse the skin, then apply a healing cream that contains zinc. Avoid all fragranced products and aromatherapy and, if you're not allergic to them, take hay fever or antihistamine tablets for three to five days.

Q. I'M BEGINNING TO SEE LINES AROUND MY LIPS. WHAT CAN I DO TO STOP THIS?

A. If you're a smoker, you can blame the dreaded cigarettes – and there's no magic wand to stop them getting worse. Try some inner mouth massage: using your thumb and forefingers, push out the skin and massage round the mouth daily (see facial yoga, chapter seven). Ensure you're using an anti-ageing serum and even a retinol product right around the mouth. Micro-needling, microcurrent and fractional radiofrequency treatments will also help.

Q. I HAVE SOME BROKEN THREAD VEINS ON MY CHEEKS. WHAT CAN I DO?

A. There isn't a product that exists to get rid of broken veins completely. They can be hereditary or related to your diet, your lifestyle and the environment you live in. A quick zap with IPL or laser will remove them. While I'm aware that lasers aren't everyone's cup of tea, treating only a small area in this way as a one-off isn't overly harsh on the skin. You can continue to use your normal skincare.

Q. I HAVE AREAS OF PIGMENTATION. IS THERE A PRODUCT THAT WILL GET RID OF IT?

A. Pigmentation is another tricky skin issue to deal with (see chapter four). Laser, peels and certain ingredients can all help, but pigment will generally bounce back if you don't have the correct skincare to prevent it.

Q. WHAT DO I NEED TO TAKE WITH ME ON MY HOLIDAY IN THE SUN?

A. Holiday packing needs to be minimal. First, stop using retinol two weeks before and don't include it again until two weeks after. If you can decant products into small bottles or pots, it saves a huge amount on weight and size. My holiday pack list is as follows:

- **Cleanser** – something that will thoroughly wash off your SPF but not over-strip skin that's been exposed to the sun.

- **SPF** – a minimum of 30 for the face.

- **Oil** – handy for cleansing, eye-make-up removal, hair nourishment, softening the cuticles, feet and facial skin.

- **A calming moisturiser** – if you get too much sun, you need something to hydrate but not irritate the skin.

- **An antioxidant serum** such as a high level vitamin C to apply under your SPF and after your shower in the evening to help fight UV damage accrued throughout the day. You'll need to keep this is in dark, airtight packaging or it'll oxidise, so it's best not to decant it.

- **A cooling spritz** – good for refreshing the skin when you're by the pool or on a flight.

- **Things to leave at home:** exfoliants, retinol-based products, anti-ageing creams, eye creams.

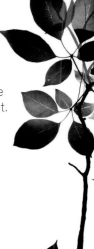

Q. I'VE NEVER HAD THE TIME TO FOLLOW A PROPER SKINCARE ROUTINE. HOW CAN I START?

A. If you have enough time to check Facebook or Instagram and watch your favourite TV series, you can easily find three minutes in the morning and in the evening for your skin. See this as you time – self-care that will benefit your mind, confidence and skin.

Q. I HAVE SENSITIVE SKIN, WHAT SHOULD I BE USING?

A. Keep it simple. Don't be fooled into thinking a hypoallergenic product is necessarily going to be the best thing for you. Organic and natural products are good, but be wary of some aromatherapy oils, which can increase sensitivity. You may need to switch your routine from time to time as your skin becomes sensitive to the products you use on a daily basis. Using a gentle milk or cream cleanser with minimal exfoliation is a great place to start.

Q. I'M 35 AND STILL USING THE SAME PRODUCTS I DID WHEN I WAS 19. IS THAT OK?

A. Some products may still be suitable, but your skin has changed in its physical structure and now needs ingredients that target its current concerns.

Q. MY SKIN LOOKS DULL. WHAT CAN I DO?

A. Ensure you're cleansing morning and night, exfoliate at least once a week and add in a mask with brightening ingredients such as AHAs or white clay. Make a home mask (see recipe on page 169 and 170) and keep it in the fridge to be used once or twice a week.

Q. DOES MY SKIN GET USED TO CERTAIN PRODUCTS AND PLATEAU?

A. No. If you've found something that works, why change it? However, there may be another product out there that works as well – if not better – for you. So there's no harm in trying something new. Just be sure to try one at a time so you can assess whether it's working or not.

Q. DO I NEED TO USE PRODUCTS FROM THE SAME SKINCARE RANGE?

A. Skincare brands usually create products that work in synergy with each other. However, the plant actives that are found in many products from different brands work together in the natural world, so there's no reason to believe they won't do so as part of your skin regimen. Just be aware of balancing your routine overall. If your cleanser contains AHAs, you may not need an exfoliant as well. Also, look out for whether both your moisturiser and serum contain retinol as together they may be too overpowering for your skin.

Q. IF I MASSAGE DOWNWARDS WILL IT SAG THE MUSCLES?

A. Your face will not sag if you massage downwards. Massaging upwards will create the best lifting effect; however the muscles and connective tissue on the face run in multiple directions, so sometimes even downwards movements are required to release tension.

Q. DO I NEED TO WEAR AN SPF EVERY DAY?

A. If you want to stave off the ageing process, then yes. The sun is the biggest premature ager and UVA rays are present all year round – not just in the summer.

Q. I CAN'T AFFORD A FACIAL. WILL MY SKIN SUFFER?

A. Be savvy with your home care and try to incorporate face massage, masks, exfoliants and kitchen cupboard remedies (see chapter nine) and you can still achieve lovely vibrant skin.

Q. I NEVER SEEM TO HAVE THE TIME TO GO FOR A FACIAL. ISN'T IT JUST SELF-INDULGENCE?

A. Don't look on a facial as a treat. We all make time for the dentist and our hairdresser and our face is what we look at every day in the mirror. Facials do wonders for your skin and sense of mental well-being.

Q. DO I REALLY NEED SO MANY PRODUCTS?

A. If you want results, collating the right wardrobe of products for you really can be a game changer.

Q. I'M GETTING MARRIED. WHEN DO I NEED TO BOOK A FACIAL?

A. Don't leave this to the last minute. Along with your dress, your face is what everyone is going to be looking at and will be photographed. If you have skin concerns such as breakouts, plan your facials at least six months before the big day. If your complexion is generally well-balanced, four months before should be sufficient. Book a course of treatments in advance. Invest in some good home care and include masks and serums as these are the powerhouses of your home regimen and will deliver great results.

Q. AT WHAT AGE DO I NEED TO START USING ANTI-AGEING PRODUCTS?

A. Our collagen production begins to slow down from the age of 25. However, I wouldn't advise investing in products labelled 'anti-ageing' until you're in your mid thirties. At 25, make sure you include antioxidants and an SPF in your home care to prevent the signs of ageing in the future.

Q. WHAT'S THE MOST COMMON MISTAKE WOMEN MAKE WHEN THEY WANT TO START USING ANTI-AGEING PRODUCTS?

A. Picking the richest cream and thinking it's going to work like magic for all their skin concerns. It's more likely to be too heavy for your skin and cause breakouts. It's better to pick the best ingredients for your skin type. I would always start by adding an antioxidant serum into your routine.

Q. WHAT'S YOUR VIEW ON FILLERS?

A. I've seen too many clients who've had a bad experience with fillers, suffering long-term complications. It's also very easy to get a distorted view of what you look like naturally if you're constantly 'correcting' perceived flaws. Often, people end up looking older because they've had so much work done.

Q. WHAT ABOUT BOTOX?

A. Botox is regularly used for important medical purposes, not just aesthetic ones. Having Botox does mean putting a toxin in your body. However, I see a lot of ladies who get to a certain age and start to become inquisitive about this treatment. If you need to try it and get it out of your system, then do. But I would suggest choosing other facial treatments to keep your complexion vibrant.

Q. WILL RUNNING MAKE MY FACE SAG?

A. No. The loss of body fat that happens when you work out regularly may cause the face to lose the appearance of plumpness, and extra sun exposure and impact of the weather might cause visible ageing, but there won't be more sagging from the physical action of running. The increase in blood flow and oxygen to the skin will make it look brighter and healthier.

Q. I KEEP GETTING REDNESS, WHAT CAN I DO?

A. Ditch the red wine and coffee; it will only make it worse. Use a gentle cleanser to freshen the skin, avoid skin wipes and toners containing alcohol and slather on a soothing mask. Try applying your mask, then placing a damp muslin cloth straight from the fridge or freezer over the top. Aloe vera is also amazing. Put it in the freezer for ten minutes, then glide it over the whole face. Check in with a skin specialist to see if you may be developing rosacea.

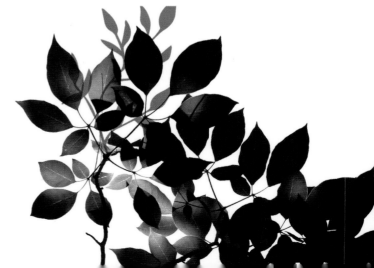

INDEX

facial acupressure 125
peels 176
repairing 145
and sleep 38
and sugar 150
and topical probiotics 117
Collagen Induction Therapy 181
colon health 122–3, 125
combination skin 75, 76, 107
contour refining 178
contraceptive pill 19, 62, 82, 89
cortisol 35, 42
cream cleansers 94
cucumber 162

D
dairy 148–9, 151
daisies 165
dandelions 165
day moisturisers 102
dehydrated skin 77
Demodex 87
Dermaroller 181
dermis 16
detoxification 42
diet 19, 21, 58, 60
digestive tract, and inflammation 142–3
dihydroxyacetone 64
dips, beauty boosting 154
DNA, damage to 35
dry skin 77, 148–9
dull skin 186

E
eczema 32, 35, 122, 142, 143, 149
elastin 16, 38
and ageing 19, 35, 66
and sugar 150
and UVA rays 26
endorphins 37, 125
enzyme peels 116, 177
epidermis 16, 176
essential fatty acids (EFAs) 54, 58, 84, 126, 144, 146
essential oils 65, 161
exercise 21, 24, 37, 71, 88, 187
exfoliation: exfoliators 15, 98, 102, 66
microdermabrasion 179

over-exfoliation 54
peels 176–7
and retinol 115
skin cycle 16
eyes: dark circles 182
de-puffing eye compress 168
eye products 41, 109
puffy eyes 182, 184
tired eye cure 168

F
face wash 94
face wipes 97
facials 58, 60, 87, 174–81, 186, 187
fair skin 81
fertile years 62
fibre 84, 141, 142
fibroblasts 16, 66
fifties, skin in your 69–71
fillers 181, 187
fish pose 48
Fitzpatrick scale 80
flavonoids 22, 146
flavonols 146, 151
flaxseeds 85, 146
flowers 165
food: foods for your skin 138–47
foods to avoid 148–51
and inflammation 142–5
link to acne 84
organic food 21
and rosacea 87
forehead 122, 125
forties, skin in your 66–8
fractional radiofrequency 181, 184, 185
free radicals 22, 112, 114, 117, 142, 144

G
gallbladder 122, 123, 125
galvanic treatments 181
gluten 148
glycolic acid 116, 177
green tea 160
gut health 138–41

H
hair, facial 60
happiness 42

happy skin hummus 154
head stand 48
heart health 122, 123, 125
herbal teas 41, 88, 160
herbs 165
high frequency treatment 181
histamines 87
holidays 185
honey 159
hormones 20–1, 125
and acne 82, 150
contraceptive pill 62
and hyperpigmentation 89
and the liver 21, 141
and stress 35, 42
see also individual hormones
hummus, happy skin 154
hyaluronic acid 66, 117
hydraquinone 117
hydrating & restoring spritz 168
hyperpigmentation 89

I
immunity 42
inflammation 138, 142–6, 149, 150–1, 166
ingredients, skincare 112–17, 159–66
insulin 35, 150
intolerances, food 149
iron 144–5
IVF 62

J
jaws 122
joint health & flexibility 42
juices, beauty boosting 153

K
keratin 52
kidneys 122, 123, 125
kojic acid 116, 177

L
lactic acid 116, 159, 161, 177
laser treatments 184, 185
laughter 37
lavender 161, 165, 184
LED light therapy 179
lemon balm 165

lifestyle 19
light brown skin 81
lighteners 166
lines, fine 19, 24, 35, 41, 185
lion pose 46
liver health 21, 122, 125, 141, 150
location, effect on skin 19
lungs 120, 122, 123, 125
lycopene 145
lymphatic system 45, 87, 131, 182

M
magnesium 21, 144, 146, 149, 151
make-up 85, 88
mandelic acid 116, 177
marigolds 165
masks 104
    balancing seaweed face mask 170
    banana peel spot treatment face mask 169
    brightening papaya pineapple face peel 169
    chocolate orange avocado nourishing mask 170
    skin restoring face mask 169
    soothing antioxidant rose petal mask 170
    spicy skin brightening mask for problem skin 170
    super greens balancing mask 170
massage 37, 41, 126–31, 174, 185, 186
matcha 146, 149
'me' time 37
meat 84, 151
medication 87, 89
meditation 32, 37, 41
melanin 26, 80, 81, 89
melanocytes 26, 89
melanoma 89
melasma 62, 64, 89
melatonin 38, 41
melting balms/oils 97
menopause 82
micellar waters 97
microcurrent therapy 178, 185
microdermabrasion 179

micro-needling 181, 184, 185
milia 86
milk cleanser 94
milk thistle 21, 141
mindfulness 32
mineral oils 54, 94
minerals 144, 146, 151
moisturisers 100–2, 166, 185
moringa 146

N
natural products 85
night creams 54, 102
normal skin 74

O
oats 160
oestrogen 20, 62, 64, 66
oils 185
    aromatherapy oils 41, 85
    essential oils 65, 161
    facial oils 41, 85, 107
    melting oils 97
oily skin 19, 52, 78, 107
olive oil 160
olive skin 81
omega-3 21, 144, 146
oranges: chocolate orange avocado nourishing mask 170
organic products 21, 87, 186
oxygen 179

P
pancreas 123, 125, 150
pansies 165
papaya 162
    brightening papaya pineapple face peel 169
peas: avocado, pea and mint dip with a kick 154
peels 15, 116, 176–7
    brightening papaya pineapple face peel 169
peptides 116
phthalates 21, 64, 82
phytoestrogens 21
pigmentation 26, 89, 117, 185
pineapple 162
    brightening papaya pineapple face peel 169

skin smoothing smoothie 153
plough pose 47
pollution 19, 22, 41
polycystic ovary disorder (PCOS) 62, 150
pore size 115, 184
potassium 146, 151
pranayama 42
prasarita padottanasana 44
prebiotics 138
pregnancy 59, 62–5, 82, 117
    and hyperpigmentation 62, 64, 89
    and retinol 114, 115
probiotics 87, 88, 117, 138, 141, 142
problem skin, spicy skin brightening mask for 170
progesterone 64
prostaglandins 149
psoriasis 32, 35, 142
psychodermatology 32
puffiness: de-puffing eye compress 168
    eyes 182, 184
    soothing face massage to beat 130–1

R
rabbit pose 44
radiofrequency (RF) 178
raspberries 162
restoring face mask, skin 169
resveratrol 112, 144
retinoids 114
retinol 114–15, 117, 143
    and milia 86
    and pregnancy 64, 115
    and skin peels 114, 177
    and sun exposure 98, 114, 115
rice flour 160
roaccutane 114
rosacea 87
    and alcohol 88, 149, 187
    and inflammation 142
    and pregnancy 64
    tips to beat 88, 87
    triggers 32, 35, 87
rose petals 165
    soothing antioxidant rose petal

With THANKS

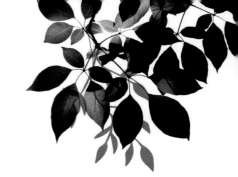

Firstly I'd like to thank all my clients whose faces I have had the privilege of treating over the years; being a therapist is a two-way relationship – hopefully improved health and skin for my clients, and increased knowledge for me.

Thank you to Adrian and Charlotte for believing in me when no other agent did.

Thank you Bella Blissett for all your 'wordy' wisdom; it would have been a jumble of words without you.

Thank you to Kyle Books who made this book happen, especially to Judith my ever patient, diplomatic and wise editor, Jenni Hare for the stunning photography, Lica Fensome for the perfect hair and makeup, beautiful every time, and Nikki Dupin for all her work on the design.

Thank you to some wise old owls for your knowledge and input: Zoe Stirling for your incredible nutritional knowledge, Hannah Whittingham for your beautiful and super-bendy yogic body, Kitty Coles for your scrummy recipes, Karen Bevan-Brown for your detailed and always thorough therapy knowledge.

Thank you to my adorable friends Cat and Sarina for always being there for me, putting a huge smile on my face and tirelessly giving feedback at every stage of this book, from concept to finish.

Thank you Melissa Hemsley for encouraging me when the process felt never ending and for generally being a beautiful bright star.

A huge hug to my three children, Georgia, James and Reuben, who have been ever patient and understanding of the crazy hours I work and a real 'A' team throughout my journey, our journey so far and for being my biggest critics, fans, inspiration and the driving force that keeps me going.

Thank you to Andrew King, George and Georgie Gordon who at earlier times in my career gave me what have turned out to be life-changing opportunities. I am forever grateful and thankful.

Thank you to the team at Liz Earle Beauty Co. who have been by my side for the past few incredible years. Special thanks to Aisling, Hannah and Leighton.

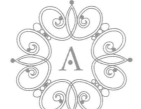

ABIGAIL JAMES

FOLLOW ABIGAIL

www.abigailjames.com

 AbigailJames1

 facebook.com/AbigailJamesLondon

 @Abigail_James